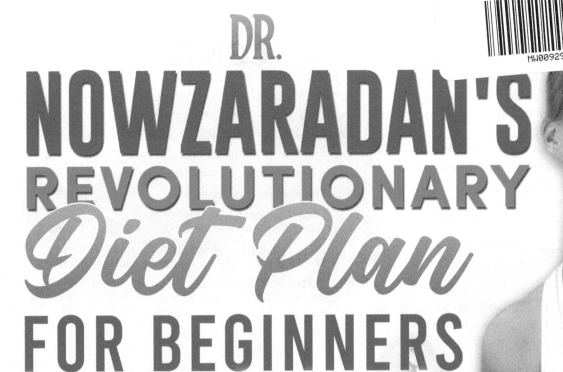

DR.
NOWZARADAN'S
REVOLUTIONARY
Diet Plan
FOR BEGINNERS
Your journey to wellness begins today

90-DAY
LOW BUDGET
MEAL PLAN

3 BONUS

FULL COLOR EDITION

2024 EDITION

EVA GOODWIN

TABLE OF CONTENTS

Chapter - 01:

INTRODUCTION TO THE "DIET BY DR. NOWZARADAN" COOKBOOK

Welcome to the transformative world of the "**Diet by Dr. Nowzaradan**," a proven pathway sculpted by the renowned Dr. Younan Nowzaradan, famously known as Dr. Now. His rigorous, medically supervised weight loss approach has not only reshaped bodies but also reinvigorated lives, especially through his pivotal role on the hit TV show "**My 600-lb Life**." Before you dive into the recipes and start your culinary journey towards a healthier you, remember: drastic weight loss processes require careful medical oversight. Therefore, **I strongly recommend that you follow these steps under the guidance of a physician and use this cookbook as a fountain of inspiration for delicious, healthful meals that align with Dr. Nowzaradan's dietary principles.**

THE MAN BEHIND THE DIET

Dr. Younan Nowzaradan, a Houston-based surgeon, ascended to prominence through his dedicated efforts in helping individuals battling severe obesity. His approach is not just about losing weight; it's a comprehensive overhaul of lifestyle and eating habits tailored to the unique medical needs of his patients. Dr. Nowzaradan's diet plan, often seen as a last resort for those who have tried almost everything else, focuses on drastically reducing calorie intake and fostering a deep understanding of nutrition and portion control.

A Benchmark for Transformative Change

On "My 600-lb Life," viewers witness the harrowing and heartwarming journeys of individuals striving to reclaim their lives from the brink of severe health crises. Under Dr. Nowzaradan's guidance, these patients learn that weight loss surgery is only a part of the equation; the real change happens in the kitchen and the mind. This is where his diet plan comes in—a meticulous, controlled-calorie diet that not only prepares individuals for surgery but sets the foundation for a sustainable, healthy lifestyle.

The Role of This Cookbook

This cookbook serves as your personal guide to navigating the complexities of a low-calorie, high-nutrition diet that has been the cornerstone of many success stories on national television. Each recipe adheres to the principles of Dr. Nowzaradan's dietary guidelines, ensuring that while the calorie count is low, the flavor and nutritional value are at their peak. Whether you are preparing for bariatric surgery or simply seeking to profoundly transform your eating habits, this cookbook is designed to provide you with a variety of meal options that align with a disciplined dietary regimen.

In these pages, you will find not just recipes but a new outlook on food—a perspective that views each meal as an opportunity to nourish, heal, and rejuvenate your body. This is not just cooking; it's a culinary journey towards recovery, health, and ultimately, a new life.

Remember, while these recipes provide a framework for healthy eating, individual needs can vary greatly. Always consult with your healthcare provider to tailor the diet plan to your specific health requirements. Use this cookbook as your culinary companion on a transformative journey that begins in the kitchen and leads to a healthier, happier you.

Objectives of the Diet: A Gateway to Transformation and Health

Welcome to a pivotal section of the "Diet by Dr. Nowzaradan" cookbook, where we dive deep into the core objectives of this rigorous dietary regimen. If you're poised on the brink of making a monumental shift in your health and lifestyle, understanding these objectives isn't just beneficial—it's crucial. The diet crafted by Dr. Nowzaradan isn't merely a set of instructions; it's a strategic blueprint designed to guide you towards significant, sustainable weight loss and optimal preparation for bariatric surgery.

Preparing for Bariatric Surgery: The First Step in a Life-Changing Journey

For many, the journey towards bariatric surgery begins with a stark realization: the need for a dramatic reduction in weight to reduce surgical risks and enhance post-operative recovery. Herein lies the first critical objective of Dr. Nowzaradan's diet—preoperative weight loss. This diet doesn't just aim to shave off pounds; it seeks to stabilize your health in a way that surgery becomes a viable, safer option.

This stringent calorie-controlled regimen is tailored to decrease body fat while preserving muscle tissue and overall nutritional status. It's about making the body a suitable candidate for surgery, ensuring that you're fortified against potential complications and primed for a successful outcome. The diet targets metabolic improvements, reduces the liver size, and decreases abdominal fat, which significantly eases the technical aspects of surgical intervention.

Sustainable Weight Loss: Beyond the Operating Room

The second, and equally vital, objective of the diet is sustainable weight loss. Dr. Nowzaradan's plan is not about quick fixes or temporary solutions. It's engineered for longevity and sustainability. Post-surgery life demands a radical transformation in eating habits and lifestyle choices. The diet sets the stage for this long-term change, embedding habits that patients need to maintain their weight loss and health improvements after surgery.

This part of the diet addresses the psychological and behavioral changes necessary for managing portion sizes, making healthier food choices, and understanding the nutritional content of meals. It's not only about losing weight but about learning a new way of life that revolves around better nutritional practices.

Controlled Dieting in a Medical Context: The Science of Eating Right

At the heart of Dr. Nowzaradan's dietary approach is the principle of controlled dieting—a meticulous, calculated method that emphasizes the importance of caloric intake and nutrient balance. This controlled approach is crucial, especially in a medical context where every calorie and nutrient has to be accounted for to meet the specific needs of the body under extreme stress from obesity.

Controlled dieting helps mitigate the risks associated with obesity, such as hypertension, diabetes, and heart disease, by fostering an environment in the body that supports health rather than detracting from it. It's a diet that's heavily backed by scientific principles, focusing on low-calorie, nutrient-dense foods that provide everything the body needs without the excessive caloric load.

The Bigger Picture: A Holistic Approach to Health

Ultimately, the diet by Dr. Nowzaradan transcends the boundaries of typical weight loss regimens. It's a holistic approach that prepares the body for a significant medical procedure and redefines the patient's relationship with food. By adhering to this diet, patients are not just striving to meet surgery criteria; they are taking the first, decisive steps towards a healthier, more active, and fulfilling life.

As you embark on this journey with the help of this cookbook, remember that each recipe and guideline is a stepping stone towards achieving these objectives. The path laid out by Dr. Nowzaradan's diet plan is comprehensive and challenging, but immensely rewarding. Armed with the right knowledge, support, and culinary inspiration from this cookbook, you are setting the stage for a profound transformation that goes well beyond the kitchen.

Chapter - 02:

PRINCIPLES OF THE DIET

Embarking on a journey toward significant weight loss and better health is no small feat—it requires a foundation built on solid, scientific dietary principles. In the "Diet by Dr. Nowzaradan," these principles are more than guidelines; they are the bedrock of a transformative process that has helped countless individuals regain control of their lives. This chapter will delve into the critical aspects of reduced caloric intake, balanced macronutrients, and the strategic reduction of sugars and carbohydrates. Each of these elements plays a pivotal role in not only achieving weight loss but ensuring it is sustainable and health-promoting in the long run.

FOUNDATIONS OF THE DIET

The diet plan developed by Dr. Nowzaradan is meticulously designed to create a caloric deficit while ensuring nutritional balance, crucial for individuals with significant weight to lose. Let's explore these foundational principles:

Reduced Caloric Intake

The Necessity of Caloric Deficit: At its core, weight loss is about energy expenditure surpassing energy intake. Dr. Nowzaradan's diet focuses on creating a caloric deficit, a scientifically proven method to trigger weight loss. By consuming fewer calories than the body burns, the diet forces the body to tap into stored fat reserves for energy, leading to weight loss.

Individual Caloric Needs: Recognizing that every individual's body and metabolic rate differ, the diet is tailored to calculate the appropriate caloric intake for each person. Factors such as age, sex, current weight, and medical conditions are considered to ensure the caloric target is both effective and safe.

Psychological and Physical Benefits: Reducing calorie intake doesn't just lead to physical weight loss; it also has significant psychological benefits. Patients often report improved mood, increased self-esteem, and a better sense of control over their lives as they make progress.

Macronutrient Balance

Roles of Macronutrients: Proteins, fats, and carbohydrates are the three main macronutrients that the body needs to function properly. Proteins are crucial for building and repairing tissues; fats provide energy and support cell growth; carbohydrates are the body's primary energy source.

Balancing for Health and Weight Loss: Dr. Nowzaradan's diet carefully balances these macronutrients to ensure optimal health while promoting weight loss. The diet is high in proteins to preserve muscle mass during the weight loss process, moderate in fats, and low in carbohydrates to avoid excessive calorie intake.

Importance of Protein: Maintaining muscle mass is crucial during weight loss. Protein-rich diets help achieve this by providing the necessary building blocks for muscle. This not only helps in keeping the metabolism active but also aids in stronger physical health as fat is lost.

Typical Meal Composition: A typical meal might include lean chicken breast (protein), a serving of steamed vegetables like broccoli or spinach (fiber and micronutrients), and a small portion of whole grains like quinoa or brown rice (complex carbohydrates).

Reduction of Sugars and Carbohydrates

Impact on Health: High intake of sugars and refined carbohydrates can lead to spikes in insulin levels, leading to increased fat storage and weight gain. Reducing these elements in the diet helps stabilize blood sugar levels and reduces the risk of diabetes and other metabolic disorders.

Craving Minimization and Fat Metabolism: By cutting down on sugars and simple carbs, the diet helps minimize cravings, making it easier for individuals to stick to their eating plan. This also enhances fat metabolism, as the body turns to stored fat for energy more frequently.

Low-Sugar and Low-Carb Alternatives: Instead of sugar-laden snacks, the diet recommends options like Greek yogurt with a handful of berries or a slice of whole-grain bread with avocado. These alternatives provide the necessary nutrients without the excessive sugars or carbs.

The principles of Dr. Nowzaradan's diet are not just about losing weight; they are about initiating a comprehensive change in how individuals consume and think about food. By adhering to these principles, patients are equipped with the tools needed for a healthier lifestyle, not just in the short term but for life.

SCIENCE OF METABOLISM

Understanding the science of metabolism is crucial in grasping how Dr. Nowzaradan's diet not only aids in significant weight loss but also in fundamentally altering the body's energy processing methods. This understanding is vital for anyone looking to undertake this diet seriously, as it provides the backbone for the dietary strategies employed.

Overview of Metabolic Processes

Metabolism at a Glance: Metabolism refers to the biochemical processes that occur within a living organism to maintain life. It's how your body converts food into energy, a complex interplay of chemical reactions that is crucial for everything from breathing to thinking to growing.

Catabolism vs. Anabolism: Within the broad spectrum of metabolism, two critical processes stand out: catabolism and anabolism. Catabolism is the breakdown of molecules to obtain energy, essentially the body's way of harvesting fuel from what you eat; it's what happens when your body digests food and breaks it down into usable energy forms. Anabolism, on the other hand, is the process of building up and using that energy to construct components of cells such as proteins and nucleic acids. Effective dieting should maintain a balance between these two processes to ensure that the body can lose weight without sacrificing muscle mass or energy levels.

Metabolic Adaptation to Weight Loss

Adapting to Lower Caloric Intake: When calories are sharply reduced, the body must adapt to using its stored energy more efficiently. Dr. Nowzaradan's diet is structured to gradually decrease caloric intake, allowing the body to adapt without triggering severe starvation responses, which can be counterproductive by slowing down the metabolism.

Changes During Weight Loss: As weight loss progresses, the body undergoes several metabolic changes. Initially, metabolism might slow down as the body attempts to conserve energy. However, with continuous adherence to the dietary adjustments, the body learns to optimize its metabolic rate to continue burning fat. This adaptive response is crucial for long-term weight loss success.

Role of the Diet in Modifying Metabolism

Optimizing Metabolic Responses: Dr. Nowzaradan's diet plan is meticulously designed to modify the body's metabolic processes to enhance fat loss. By adjusting macronutrient intake and reducing calorie consumption, the diet prompts the body to favor fat burning over carbohydrate reliance.

Metabolic Flexibility: One of the cornerstones of this diet is enhancing metabolic flexibility—the body's ability to switch between burning carbs and fats efficiently. This flexibility is crucial for those undergoing significant weight loss as it allows the body to adapt to different energy sources based on dietary intake and activity levels.

Enhancing Metabolic Efficiency

Boosting Metabolism Through Diet and Lifestyle Changes: The timing of meals can significantly affect metabolic rate. Dr. Nowzaradan's diet includes recommendations for regular meal times, which help maintain a steady metabolic rate throughout the day. Furthermore, integrating specific types of exercise, particularly strength training, can increase muscle mass, thereby boosting metabolic rate since muscle burns more calories than fat.

Importance of Hydration and Micronutrients: Proper hydration is essential for optimizing metabolism. Water is crucial for processing calories, so even mild dehydration can slow down metabolism. Additionally, micronutrients play vital roles in various metabolic pathways; deficiencies can disrupt metabolic balance. This diet ensures adequate intake of essential vitamins and minerals to support metabolic health, encouraging consumption of nutrient-dense foods that provide these vital substances.

The science of metabolism as it relates to Dr. Nowzaradan's diet underscores a profound understanding of how the body processes, utilizes, and stores energy. By following the principles laid out in this diet, individuals can harness these metabolic processes to not only lose significant weight but also improve their overall metabolic health, leading to a healthier, more energetic life.

As we wrap up this enlightening journey through the foundational principles of the "Diet by Dr. Nowzaradan," it's crucial to revisit and cement the core concepts that make this diet not just a plan, but a gateway to a transformed life. We've delved deep into the intricacies of reduced caloric intake, balanced macronutrients, and the strategic reduction of sugars and carbohydrates. Each of these elements is not just a piece of the puzzle in isolation; together, they create a powerful synergy that drives substantial weight loss and enhances metabolic health.

Understanding the dynamics of metabolism—how it can be manipulated through diet to switch between burning fats and carbohydrates, and how it can be optimized through proper meal timing and micronutrient intake—empowers us. It's not just about losing weight; it's about fostering a metabolic environment that promotes sustained health and vitality.

Chapter - 03:

MEAL PLANNING GUIDE

Embarking on Dr. Nowzaradan's diet isn't just about choosing to eat less; it's about choosing to eat right. Successful implementation of this diet hinges on meticulous meal planning—a disciplined approach that not only guides you toward your weight loss goals but also enhances your overall metabolic health. Structured meal planning transforms random eating into a deliberate strategy to control calorie intake while ensuring each meal is nutritionally balanced. This foundation not only facilitates effective weight loss but also establishes habits that foster long-term health and well-being. In this chapter, we'll explore the intricacies of meal organization, offering practical insights and examples to help you master the art of meal planning within the caloric confines of Dr. Nowzaradan's renowned diet.

MEAL ORGANIZATION

Understanding Caloric Limits

- **Determining Your Caloric Boundary:** The first step in adhering to Dr. Nowzaradan's diet plan is to understand your unique caloric needs. This determination is based on various factors, including age, gender, current weight, metabolic health, and activity level. Tools such as metabolic rate calculators or consultations with a healthcare provider can offer a personalized caloric target that aligns with your weight loss objectives.

- **The Importance of Compliance:** Sticking to your caloric limits is paramount for the success of the diet. It's not merely about reducing food intake but about adhering to a calculated regimen that maximizes fat loss while preserving muscle mass and ensuring nutritional adequacy.

Structuring Your Daily Menus

- **Dividing Daily Intake:** A well-organized daily menu divides the total caloric allowance across meals and snacks in a way that sustains energy levels and manages hunger. Typically, this could involve allocating specific calorie portions to breakfast, lunch, dinner, and one or two snacks.

- **Planning for Balance and Satiety:** Each meal should be planned to balance macronutrients—proteins, fats, and carbohydrates—to optimize nutrition and satiety. High-protein breakfasts, fiber-rich lunches, balanced dinners, and nutrient-dense snacks can help manage cravings and avoid overeating.

Sample Daily Menus

Example 1: 1200 Calorie/Day Plan
- **Breakfast:** Greek yogurt with mixed berries and a sprinkle of flaxseed (300 calories)
- **Lunch:** Grilled chicken salad with mixed greens, cherry tomatoes, and vinaigrette (350 calories)
- **Dinner:** Broiled salmon with steamed broccoli and quinoa (400 calories)
- **Snack:** Carrot sticks with hummus (150 calories)

Example 2: 1500 Calorie/Day Plan
- **Breakfast:** Oatmeal with sliced almonds and banana (350 calories)
- **Lunch:** Turkey and avocado wrap with whole grain tortilla and side salad (450 calories)
- **Dinner:** Beef stir-fry with bell peppers, broccoli, and brown rice (500 calories)
- **Snack:** An apple with peanut butter (200 calories)

Adjusting Menus According to Personal Preferences and Nutritional Needs

- **Food Swapping for Personalization:** Flexibility within dietary confines is crucial for maintaining long-term adherence. Swapping foods within similar caloric and macronutrient profiles allows you to cater to personal taste preferences and prevent diet fatigue without compromising the diet's effectiveness.

- **Maintaining Dietary Flexibility:** While the diet sets strict caloric boundaries, it allows for adjustments based on individual responses and changes in dietary needs. This flexibility can be crucial for addressing nutritional deficiencies, adapting to changes in physical activity, or managing medical conditions.

Successful meal planning on Dr. Nowzaradan's diet requires understanding and respecting your caloric limits, structuring your meals to maintain balance and satiety, and adapting the diet to fit your personal preferences and nutritional needs. By mastering these aspects, you can turn Dr. Nowzaradan's principles into a practical, everyday lifestyle that promotes significant weight loss and enhances metabolic health.

PORTION CONTROL

In the journey to significant weight loss, one of the most critical strategies is mastering portion control. This skill is essential not only for achieving your initial weight loss goals but also for maintaining that success long-term. Portion control directly impacts your caloric intake, which is the linchpin of Dr. Nowzaradan's diet plan. By managing portions, you ensure that you consume the right amount of calories without overeating, regardless of the type of food you choose.

The principle is straightforward: if you can control your portions, you can control your calories and thus your weight. Accurate portion control allows for a flexible diet that can adapt to different settings and situations, making weight management a practical part of daily life rather than a constant struggle.

Techniques for Measuring Portions

- **Using Kitchen Scales for Precision:** The most effective way to ensure you are eating the correct portion sizes is to use a kitchen scale. A scale removes the guesswork from portion control, providing you with the exact weight of your food. For those following Dr. Nowzaradan's diet, where every calorie must be accounted for, a kitchen scale becomes an indispensable tool in your culinary arsenal.

- **Estimating Portion Sizes with Household Items:** Not everyone has access to a kitchen scale at every meal, especially when dining out. Learning to estimate portion sizes using common household items can be incredibly helpful. For example, a single serving of meat (3 ounces) is about the size of a deck of cards, a cup of pasta is roughly the size of a tennis ball, and an ounce of cheese is about the size of a pair of dice. These visual cues help you stay within your dietary limits, even when you can't measure portions precisely.

Tools for Portion Control

- **Essential Portion Control Tools:** Beyond kitchen scales, other tools can help maintain portion control. Measuring cups and spoons are perfect for accurately serving sizes of liquids and powders. For solid foods that fit into them, like rice or chopped vegetables, they're equally useful.

- **Benefits of Utilizing Portion Control Tools:** Using these tools consistently helps inculcate a habit of mindfulness about the quantity of food you consume. It trains your eye to recognize correct portion sizes and your mind to understand how much food is enough, thereby helping avoid the common pitfall of overeating.

Practical Tips for Portion Control

Understanding Food Labels: One of the keys to effective portion control is understanding food labels correctly. Every label provides serving size information, but it's crucial to note that a package might contain more than one serving.

Misinterpreting food labels can lead to unintentional overeating. By becoming proficient in reading these labels, you can better manage your intake according to the diet's guidelines.

Strategies for Eating Out: Dining out can be a challenge when you're trying to adhere to a strict diet plan. Here are a few strategies to manage portion control in social settings:

- Ask for half-portions or a children's menu size if available.
- Share a meal with someone else to avoid oversized restaurant portions.
- Request a box at the beginning of your meal and place half of it to take home for another meal.
- Choose side dishes wisely—opt for salads or steamed vegetables instead of fries or creamy sides.
- These strategies empower you to enjoy social occasions without straying from your meal plan, ensuring that your dietary efforts are consistent and effective, no matter the setting.

Portion control is not just a diet tactic; it is a lifestyle change that promotes better eating habits and a healthier relationship with food. By mastering the methods and tools of portion control, you set yourself up for success in both losing weight and maintaining a healthy weight for life, fully embracing the principles of Dr. Nowzaradan's dietary guidance.

TAKEAWAY

As we close this chapter on meal planning and portion control within the framework of Dr. Nowzaradan's diet plan, it's crucial to revisit and emphasize the core principles that can drive your success in this transformative journey. Effective meal planning and stringent portion control are not merely suggestions; they are essential strategies that lay the foundation for achieving and maintaining significant weight loss.

Structured Meal Planning: By planning your meals meticulously—accounting for caloric limits, ensuring nutritional balance, and preparing for each day—you arm yourself against common diet pitfalls such as impulsive eating and dietary monotony. Remember, a well-laid plan is your first step towards success.

Rigorous Portion Control: Mastering portion control allows you to maintain strict adherence to the caloric goals set forth by Dr. Nowzaradan's diet. Whether it's by using scales, measuring cups, or visual comparisons, knowing how much to eat plays a pivotal role in controlling your caloric intake effectively.

Consistency is Key: These strategies require consistent application. It's not about being perfect for a day but about being diligent every day. The consistency of your efforts will determine the consistency of your results. Each day that you stick to your plan, you build habits that not only facilitate weight loss but also help maintain it in the long run.

Moving Forward: Embrace the power of these meal planning and portion control strategies as a way to reclaim control over your diet and, by extension, your health. This is more than a diet; it's a new way of life—a life where you have the power to shape your future through informed and mindful choices about what you eat.

Let this chapter serve as a cornerstone upon which you build a healthier, more vibrant life. Remember, the journey to weight loss is not a sprint; it's a marathon. Each step you take with discipline and awareness brings you closer to your ultimate goal of health and wellness. Stay the course, remain committed, and watch as you transform not only your body but also your confidence and quality of life.

Chapter - 04:

MANAGING EXPECTATIONS AND THE PSYCHOLOGY OF CHANGE

In Dr. Nowzaradan's diet plan, weight loss is more than just following nutritional guidelines - it is a profound transformation that involves both body and mind. It's essential to understand from the outset that successful weight management is as much about managing expectations and mastering psychological challenges as it is about following dietary prescriptions. Realistic goal-setting and psychological resilience form the bedrock of this transformative journey.

Setting realistic goals is not about tempering ambition but about crafting a vision that is achievable and sustainable over the long term. This approach helps prevent the common pitfalls of frustration and burnout, which can derail even the most dedicated efforts. Similarly, psychological resilience—the ability to bounce back from setbacks and maintain a positive outlook—is indispensable. Weight loss is rarely linear; there will be hurdles, plateaus, and days when motivation wanes. Here, the right mental approach can make the difference between a setback that ends your journey and one that strengthens your resolve.

As we delve deeper into this chapter, we'll explore how you can set practical, achievable goals and strategies to enhance your psychological resilience. By understanding the emotional and cognitive aspects of dietary change, you'll be equipped not only to start your journey with a robust plan but also to continue with the perseverance and adaptability needed to see it through to success. This dual focus on the practical and the psychological is what transforms a diet plan from a mere regimen to a sustainable lifestyle change, leading to lasting health and wellness.

REALISTIC EXPECTATIONS

Choosing Dr. Nowzaradan's diet plan means embarking on a journey of discipline and change. But the keystone to navigating this path successfully is setting realistic expectations—a crucial step that ensures sustained effort, reduces disappointment and maximizes your success potential. This section delves into how you can set achievable goals, understand the typical timelines for weight loss, and find joy in celebrating milestones, all tailored to your unique journey.

Setting Realistic Goals

The importance of setting achievable goals cannot be overstated. Goals that are too ambitious may lead to disappointment and a quick burnout, while goals that are too modest may not provide enough challenge to keep you engaged. To find that perfect balance, you need to consider your starting point and personal circumstances—your current weight, health conditions, and lifestyle all play critical roles in determining what's achievable for you.

Begin by consulting with a healthcare provider to understand your physical constraints and get a baseline of your health metrics. Next, set short-term and long-term goals. For instance, a short-term goal could be to follow the diet strictly for one month, and a long-term goal could be to reach a weight loss milestone in six months. Remember, realistic goals are SMART: Specific, Measurable, Achievable, Relevant, and Time-bound.

Timelines for Weight Loss

Understanding and accepting typical timelines for weight loss can help adjust your expectations and keep you motivated. Weight loss with Dr. Nowzaradan's diet is gradual. Rapid weight loss is not sustainable and can be detrimental to your health. Most individuals on this plan can expect to lose weight at a rate determined by their metabolic rate, adherence to the dietary regimen, and initial body weight.

It's crucial to monitor your progress and adjust your expectations based on your health changes. If you have a month where you don't lose as much as expected, evaluate what adjustments might be necessary—whether in calorie intake, meal planning, or physical activity—but also recognize that plateaus are a normal part of the weight loss process.

Celebrating Milestones

Recognizing and celebrating milestones is vital for maintaining morale on your weight loss journey. These celebrations can reinforce your commitment to your goals and refresh your motivation. However, it's important to find ways to celebrate that do not involve food, which can counteract your progress.

Instead, consider rewards like a new workout outfit, a day off for some personal pampering, or a new book. Another effective celebration is to share your successes with friends or a support group who will celebrate with you and encourage you to continue. Additionally, documenting your journey through photos or a journal can provide tangible evidence of your progress, offering a boost of confidence when needed.

PSYCHOLOGICAL CHALLENGES

Transitioning to a new diet, especially one as structured as Dr. Nowzaradan's, is not just a physical challenge but a deeply psychological one. The journey to significant weight loss involves more than just changing what you eat; it fundamentally alters your relationship with food. This section addresses the psychological hurdles you may encounter, strategies to overcome internal resistance, and ways to maintain a positive outlook through the ups and downs of your weight loss journey.

Understanding the Challenges of Changing Eating Habits

Changing eating habits is a profound psychological challenge, often underpinned by deeply ingrained behaviors and emotional connections with food. Common hurdles include cravings for unhealthy foods, emotional eating in response to stress or sadness, and automatic behaviors—such as eating while watching TV—that have become habitual over years. These challenges are formidable but not insurmountable.

The role of mindset in this transformation cannot be overstated. Viewing these changes as positive, life-enhancing adjustments rather than punitive measures can dramatically affect your ability to stick to the new diet. Educating yourself about the nutritional aspects of food and the detrimental impacts of unhealthy eating can also reinforce your commitment to change.

Overcoming Internal Resistance

Resistance to change is a natural psychological reaction; your mind tends to revert to known patterns under stress or uncertainty. Cognitive behavioral strategies can be highly effective in combating this. These involve identifying negative thought patterns that lead to unhealthy eating behaviors and systematically replacing them with positive ones. Mindfulness practices help you stay present and aware, reducing impulsive eating, while stress management techniques such as deep breathing, yoga, or even regular physical exercise can reduce the emotional need to find comfort in food. Consistency in these practices cultivates a new normal for your psyche, slowly reducing the internal resistance you might feel. Setting small, manageable goals can help maintain motivation and make the process feel less overwhelming.

Maintaining a Positive Attitude

The path to weight loss is rarely linear, and setbacks are a normal part of any journey. Staying positive during these times is crucial. Reframe setbacks as learning opportunities and remember that every day is a chance to restart with renewed vigor. Keeping a gratitude journal where you record not just your diet and exercise but also things you are grateful for each day can shift your focus from what you're missing to what you're gaining.

Building resilience is easier with a supportive environment. Lean on friends, family, or join support groups where you can share experiences and strategies with others on similar journeys. Professional guidance from a psychologist or a counselor skilled in behavioral change can also provide tools to manage the psychological aspects of weight loss effectively.

STRATEGIES FOR LONG-TERM SUCCESS

Achieving your weight loss goals through Dr. Nowzaradan's diet plan is only the beginning. The true challenge—and victory—lies in maintaining those results over the long term. This requires not just a temporary change, but a permanent adjustment in both behavior and mindset. Here, we explore essential strategies for sustained weight management and psychological tools that can support you throughout this enduring journey.

Behavioral Adjustments for Sustained Weight Management

Embracing Flexible Dieting: One of the most effective strategies for long-term dietary success is flexible dieting. This approach allows for a more moderate variation in your eating habits, which can include planned indulgences. The key is to balance these moments with healthier choices throughout your day, ensuring that you stay within your caloric goals while still enjoying life's culinary pleasures.

Integrating Intermittent Fasting: Intermittent fasting (IF) is another strategy that can be integrated into your long-term plan. IF focuses not on what you eat but when you eat, establishing eating windows that help control calorie intake and enhance metabolic health. For example, the 16/8 method, where you eat during an 8-hour window and fast for 16 hours, can be a sustainable approach if it fits your lifestyle and medical conditions.

Tips for Daily Integration:

- **Plan Your Meals:** Use meal planning as a tool to prevent last-minute decision-making, which often leads to less healthy choices.

- **Cook in Bulk:** Prepare and store multiple meals at once to alleviate the daily burden of cooking.

- **Healthy Swaps:** Develop a repertoire of healthy substitutions for high-calorie favorites to avoid feelings of deprivation.

Psychological Tools and Resources

Utilizing Psychological Tools: The psychological challenges of maintaining weight loss are often as daunting as the dietary adjustments themselves. Tools such as cognitive-behavioral therapy (CBT) can help you develop healthier eating habits and combat negative thought patterns. Mindfulness meditation is another effective tool that enhances your awareness of hunger and satiety cues, helping you make conscious food choices.

Leveraging Resources: Numerous resources can aid your journey, including:

Support Groups: Whether online or in-person, support groups provide a community of individuals facing similar challenges, offering an environment of encouragement and understanding.

Motivational Books and Apps: Books that promote positive psychology and apps that track dietary intake and exercise can motivate you to stay on course.

Professional Guidance: Regular consultations with a dietitian or a psychologist can provide personalized strategies and support.

Benefits of Ongoing Mental Health Support:

1. **Addressing Underlying Issues:** Mental health professionals can help uncover and address emotional or psychological issues related to eating behaviors.

2. **Developing Coping Strategies:** Learn coping mechanisms for stress, anxiety, or depression that don't involve food.

3. **Reinforcing Positive Changes:** Continuous psychological support helps reinforce the lifestyle changes necessary for long-term success, ensuring these new habits become ingrained.

TAKEAWAY

As we conclude this chapter on managing expectations and the psychology of change, it's crucial to underscore the importance of setting realistic goals and utilizing psychological tools. These elements are foundational for successful, sustained weight management. Remember, the journey you are embarking on with Dr. Nowzaradan's diet plan is not solely about the foods you eat but also about fundamentally understanding and reshaping your habits and behaviors.

Take advantage of the power of positive thinking and self-compassion throughout your journey. It's normal to encounter setbacks, but the resilience to overcome them is built on a positive mindset and an understanding attitude towards oneself. Each step forward, no matter how small, is a part of your progress. Celebrate these moments, learn from the challenges, and persist with determination. Recognize that changing your diet is as much a mental endeavor as it is a physical one. Mastering the psychological aspects of this change is as crucial as adhering to the nutritional guidelines. By integrating both, you equip yourself for not just temporary success, but for achieving and maintaining your health goals over the long term. Keep focused, stay motivated, and remember that this journey is about creating a healthier, happier you.

Chapter - 05:

TIPS FOR LONG-TERM SUCCESS

Achieving weight loss is a monumental achievement, yet the true victory lies in maintaining those results over the long haul. Long-term success in weight management demands more than transient enthusiasm; it requires a deep-seated commitment to sustained lifestyle changes and the continuous application of learned principles. This journey, while challenging, is immensely rewarding, offering not only continued health benefits but also a renewed sense of self-confidence and control.

We delve into the crucial strategies that help maintain your weight loss success and prevent the dreaded rebound. From practical advice on navigating high-temptation situations to adopting routine behaviors that fortify your new lifestyle, we will cover all you need to stay on track. Additionally, we will explore inspirational testimonials from individuals who have triumphed over their weight struggles by adhering to Dr. Nowzaradan's diet. These stories not only prove the diet's effectiveness but also provide the motivational boost to keep pushing forward. This chapter is designed to equip you with the tools and inspiration needed for enduring success through a combination of steadfast maintenance strategies and compelling success narratives.

MAINTENANCE STRATEGIES

Maintaining long-term weight loss is an ongoing process that demands more than just initial success; it requires a lifelong commitment to healthful practices and thoughtful decision-making. In this section, we'll delve into effective strategies for continuing your weight loss journey, preventing weight regain, and establishing routines that foster sustained success. Whether you're navigating daily choices or special challenges, the following strategies will help you maintain your achievements and continue improving your health.

Continuing Weight Loss

For many, the end of an intense weight loss phase isn't the end of the journey. Continuing to lose weight in a slow, steady manner can be crucial for those with significant goals. It's important to focus on sustainable habits rather than quick fixes:

- **Adjusting Caloric Intake:** As your weight decreases, so does your caloric need. Regularly recalibrating your caloric intake is crucial to match your body's changing energy expenditure.
- **Increasing Physical Activity:** As you become fitter, your body becomes more efficient at burning calories, which might require you to increase the intensity or duration of your workouts to avoid plateaus.
- **Setting New, Small Goals:** Keep yourself motivated by setting mini-goals that are achievable and measurable. These can be related to behavior (e.g., walking 10,000 steps a day) or outcomes (e.g., losing 5 pounds in a month).

Preventing Weight Regain

Maintaining weight loss is often harder than losing it. Here are some strategies to prevent slipping back into old habits:

- **Identify Triggers:** Learn to recognize the situations that make you prone to overeating—stress, social pressures, emotional distress—and develop strategies to cope with them without turning to food.
- **Plan for Temptations:** Plan your meals ahead of time during holidays, vacations, and social gatherings. Decide what you'll eat and what you'll avoid, and stick to your plan.
- **Mindful Eating:** Stay conscious of each bite during meals. This practice helps you enjoy your food more and recognize when you are full.

Daily Routines and Habits

The establishment of daily routines can significantly influence your long-term weight management success:

- **Consistent Meal Times:** Eat at regular times to prevent overeating and keep your metabolism steady.
- **Meal Prepping:** Prepare meals in advance to avoid making impulsive food choices when you're hungry.
- **Regular Exercise:** Incorporate physical activity into your daily routine, whether it's a morning jog, yoga, or a post-dinner walk.
- **Adequate Sleep:** Ensure you get at least 7-8 hours of sleep per night, as lack of sleep can lead to weight gain.

Nutritional Adjustments

As your lifestyle changes, so too should your diet. Continuous adjustments will ensure it remains aligned with your health needs and weight goals:

- **Periodic Reviews:** Regularly review your eating habits to ensure they still meet your nutritional needs as your body and activities change.
- **Balanced Diet:** Ensure your diet remains balanced with a good mix of proteins, carbohydrates, and fats. Adjust the ratios as needed based on your current health and activity levels.
- **Hydration:** Never underestimate the importance of staying hydrated. Water helps control appetite and maintain metabolism.

TESTIMONIALS

The journey to sustained weight loss is often punctuated by stories of personal triumph and transformative change. These real-life success stories not only serve to motivate and inspire but also provide tangible proof of what is achievable with dedication, the right strategies, and a commitment to Dr. Nowzaradan's diet plan. In this section, we'll explore detailed testimonials from individuals who have not only lost significant weight but have also maintained their new, healthier lifestyles over the long term.

Success Story 1: John's Journey

John, a 45-year-old office worker, faced severe health warnings due to his weight. After starting Dr. Nowzaradan's diet, John learned to manage his calorie intake meticulously and incorporated walking into his daily routine. Over two years, he lost over 150 pounds. The biggest change for John was in his approach to eating; he adopted meal prepping and mindful eating, which he credits for his ability to maintain his current weight. His journey shows the importance of integrating simple, daily exercises and consistent meal habits into one's life.

Success Story 2: Maria's Transformation

Maria, a mother of three, struggled with postpartum weight gain that spiraled into emotional eating. Her turning point came when she began following the structured meal plans and nutritional guidance of Dr. Nowzaradan's diet. By setting incremental goals, celebrating small victories, and using support groups for motivation, Maria gradually lost 100 pounds. Today, she is not only more active but also volunteers as a mentor to others starting their weight loss journeys. Her story underscores the power of community support and setting achievable, step-by-step goals.

Lessons Learned

John and Maria teach valuable lessons about the power of persistence and the importance of incorporating manageable lifestyle changes. Their successes exemplify how effectively applying the maintenance strategies discussed earlier—such as meal prepping, mindful eating, and community support—can lead to sustainable weight loss and a healthier life overall. These testimonials are a testament to the fact that while the path to weight loss is personal and can be challenging, it is also laden with victories that can inspire others to embark on or continue their journeys. Each story not only motivates but also lights the way for new adherents of the diet, providing real-world examples of how the principles and strategies of Dr. Nowzaradan's diet can be successfully applied to achieve and maintain significant weight loss.

ENCOURAGEMENT AND MOTIVATION

Weight loss is an exciting yet often daunting endeavor. As you progress, it's natural for initial bursts of motivation to ebb, making it increasingly difficult to stay on track. Understanding how to nurture your motivation and keep your commitment strong is essential for long-term success. In this section, we'll delve into the dynamics of maintaining motivation, renewing your commitment when it falters, and embracing the ongoing journey of learning and adapting your lifestyle.

The Role of Motivation in Long-Term Success

Motivation is the fuel that drives the journey to weight loss, but unlike a simple tank of gas, it requires continuous replenishment. It's normal for your motivation levels to fluctuate due to various factors like changes in routine, emotional stresses, or even significant milestones reached. Recognizing that these fluctuations are part of the process allows you to manage them proactively. Sustaining high motivation over time is key; it involves setting clear, achievable goals and regularly reminding yourself why you started this journey in the first place. Keeping your eye on the ultimate prize with a positive mindset helps you overcome the inevitable ups and downs along the way.

Renewing Commitment

There will be days when your initial resolve may waver and when the goals seem just out of reach. During these times, renewing your commitment becomes crucial:

- **Revisit Your 'Why':** Regularly remind yourself of the reasons you started your weight loss journey. Whether it's for health, improved self-esteem, or for your loved ones, reconnecting with your why can reignite your motivation.

- **Set New Goals:** As you achieve your initial goals, set new ones to keep your journey challenging and engaging. These goals don't always have to be about weight loss; they can be about fitness levels, dietary milestones, or mental health improvements.

- **Seek Support:** Never underestimate the power of a supportive community. Whether it's friends, family, or an online support group, shared experiences and encouragement can boost your motivation immensely.

Continuous Learning and Adaptation

Approach your weight loss journey as a lifelong learning experience. The body you have today is not the one you will have a year from now, and your needs, capabilities, and challenges will change:

- **Stay Informed:** Keep up-to-date with the latest nutritional research and advice that can help refine and optimize your diet plan.

- **Listen to Your Body:** Pay attention to how your body responds to different foods, exercises, and lifestyle changes. What works well one month might not work the next.

- Adjust your diet and exercise plans based on what your body tells you.

- **Embrace Flexibility:** Flexibility in your approach can help you manage unexpected situations without derailing your progress. Adapt your meal plans and workouts to fit changes in your schedule or lifestyle.

TAKEAWAY

As we conclude this chapter on achieving and maintaining long-term success, it's vital to reflect on the core strategies that pave the way for a sustained transformation. This journey, as exemplified by the inspirational testimonials shared, is not just about reaching a target weight but about continuously setting and achieving new health and wellness goals throughout your life. Embrace the maintenance strategies that have been outlined—strategically adjusting your diet, staying vigilant against weight regain, and embedding healthful routines into your daily life. Remember, the journey of weight loss is profoundly personal and ever-evolving. As you adapt and learn, your ability to maintain your achievements will strengthen.

Part 2:
COOKBOOK

CELEBRATING CULINARY DIVERSITY

In this section of our cookbook, we embark on a delightful culinary journey that bridges the diverse and rich food traditions of America and Britain. The goal is to celebrate the wide array of cooking styles, ingredients, and tastes that each culture offers, while also introducing readers to different culinary variants. This approach not only enriches the dining experience but also encourages a deeper appreciation for how regional influences can transform a simple meal into something uniquely flavorful and memorable.

We invite you to explore these recipes with an open mind and adventurous spirit. Whether you prefer the hearty, comforting touch typical of American cuisine or the refined, aromatic flavors characteristic of British fare, there's something here to expand your culinary horizons. Each recipe includes options for adding an "American Touch" or a "British Touch," allowing you to customize dishes according to your taste or curiosity about international flavors.

RDV = RECOMMENDED DAILY VALUE

The RDV, or Recommended Daily Value, refers to the guideline amounts of nutrients that a person should consume daily based on public health recommendations. These values are set by health authorities and are intended to help consumers understand the nutritional content of their food in relation to a total daily diet. The RDV is often used on food and dietary supplement labeling to indicate the percentage of the recommended daily amount of each nutrient that a serving of the food provides. It's an essential tool for guiding individuals in maintaining a balanced diet and ensuring they receive adequate levels of essential nutrients each day. This is particularly useful when managing dietary needs, preventing nutritional deficiencies, and promoting overall health.

1. SPINACH AND BLUEBERRY PROTEIN SMOOTHIE

 Prep time: 5 minutes   **Cooking time:** Not Expected   **Total time:** 5 minutes   **Servings:** 1

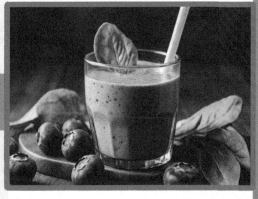

Ingredients
- **Fresh spinach:** 1 cup (30 g)
- **Frozen blueberries:** 1/2 cup (70 g)
- **Sugar-free protein powder:** 1 scoop (about 30 g)
- **Unsweetened almond milk:** 1 cup (240 ml)

American Touch:
- **Avocado:** ¼ (50g)

British Touch:
- **Elderberry or blackcurrant jam:** 1 tbsp

Step-by-Step Instructions
1. **Combine Ingredients:** In a blender, combine the fresh spinach, frozen blueberries, protein powder, and almond milk.
   - **American Touch:** For an American twist, add ¼ of an avocado to the mixture.
   - **British Touch:** For a British touch, add 1 tbsp of elderberry or blackcurrant jam.
2. **Blend:** Blend on high speed until the mixture is smooth and creamy.
3. **Adjust Flavor:** Taste and, if necessary, add a sweetener of your choice to reach the desired sweetness.
4. **Serve:** Pour the smoothie into a tall glass and consume immediately to enjoy its nutritional properties at their best.

Tips and Variations
- **More Fiber:** Add a tsp of chia or flax seeds for an extra fiber boost.
- **Extra Flavor:** For an added touch of flavor, try adding a pinch of vanilla extract or ground cinnamon.

Storage and Serving Suggestions
- **Freshness:** This smoothie is best consumed immediately but can be stored in the refrigerator for up to 24 hours. Shake well before drinking if it has been refrigerated.

Nutritional Information per Serving
- **Calories:** 200 kcal
- **Protein:** 15 g (30% of RDV)
- **Carbohydrates:** 25 g (9%)
- **Sugars:** 12 g
- **Fat:** 5 g (8%)
- **Saturated Fat:** 0.5 g (2.5%)
- **Fiber:** 4 g (16%)
- **Sodium:** 150 mg (6.5%)

2. HERB OMELETTE WITH BELL PEPPERS

 Prep time: 10 minutes   **Cooking time:** 5 minutes   **Total time:** 15 minutes   **Servings:** 1

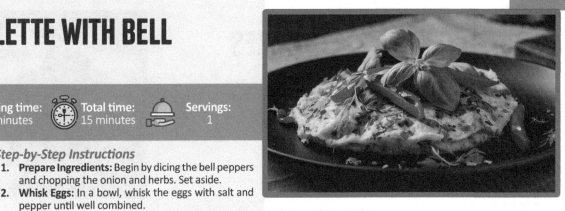

Ingredients
- **Eggs:** 3 large
- **Red bell peppers:** 1, finely diced
- **Onion:** 1 small, finely chopped
- **Fresh herbs (basil, parsley):** 1/4 cup, chopped
- **Salt:** 1/4 tsp, or to taste
- **Pepper:** 1/4 tsp, or to taste

American Touch:
- **Low-fat cheese or dairy-free cheese alternative:** 1/4 cup, grated

British Touch:
- **Turmeric:** 1/2 tsp

Step-by-Step Instructions
1. **Prepare Ingredients:** Begin by dicing the bell peppers and chopping the onion and herbs. Set aside.
2. **Whisk Eggs:** In a bowl, whisk the eggs with salt and pepper until well combined.
   - **British Touch:** Add 1/2 tsp of turmeric to the eggs for a vibrant color and a hint of earthy flavor.
   - **American Touch:** Stir in the grated low-fat cheese or dairy-free cheese alternative to the egg mixture for a creamy texture and rich flavor.
3. **Cook Vegetables:** Heat a non-stick skillet over medium heat. Add a small amount of oil or butter, then sauté the onions and bell peppers until they are soft, about 3-4 minutes.
4. **Add Herbs and Eggs:** Reduce the heat to low, add the chopped herbs to the skillet, and pour the egg mixture over the sautéed vegetables.
5. **Cook Omelette:** Allow the eggs to cook undisturbed until the edges start to lift from the skillet. Use a spatula to gently lift the edges and tilt the pan to let uncooked egg flow underneath.
6. **Fold and Serve:** Once the omelette is set but still slightly runny on top, fold it in half and slide it onto a plate. Serve immediately.

Tips and Variations
- **Add More Vegetables:** Feel free to include additional vegetables like spinach or mushrooms for extra flavor and nutrients.
- **Spice It Up:** A dash of chili flakes can add a spicy kick to the omelette.

Storage and Serving Suggestions
- **Freshness:** This dish is best enjoyed fresh. If necessary, it can be stored in the refrigerator for up to 24 hours and reheated gently.

Nutritional Information per Serving
- **Calories:** 300 kcal - **Protein:** 20 g (40% of RDV)
- **Carbohydrates:** 10 g (4% of RDV)
- **Sugars:** 4 g (no daily recommended value for added sugars)
- **Fat:** 20 g (31% of RDV) - **Saturated Fat:** 5 g (25% of RDV)
- **Fiber:** 2 g (8% of RDV) - **Sodium:** 400 mg (17% of RDV)

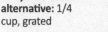

3. GREEK YOGURT WITH NUTS

 Prep time: 5 minutes   **Cooking time:** Not Expected   **Total time:** 5 minutes   **Servings:** 1

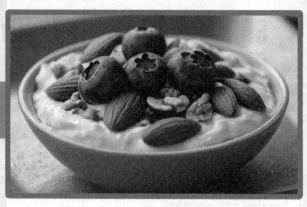

Ingredients

- **Non-fat Greek yogurt:** 1 cup (245 g)
- **Chopped nuts (such as almonds, walnuts, or pecans):** 1/4 cup (30 g)
- **Cinnamon:** 1/2 tsp

American Touch:

- **Blueberries:** 1/4 cup (37 g)
- **Sugar-free granola:** 2 tbsps (14 g)

British Touch:

- **Sugar-free blackcurrant jam:** 1 tbsp (20 g)

Step-by-Step Instructions

1. **Prepare the Base:** In a serving bowl, add 1 cup of non-fat Greek yogurt. Sprinkle with cinnamon and add the chopped nuts, mixing slightly to combine.

   - **Add the American Touch:** For an American twist, top the yogurt with fresh blueberries and a sprinkle of sugar-free granola for added texture and sweetness.
   - **Add the British Touch:** For a British variant, stir in a tbsp of sugar-free blackcurrant jam, swirling it through the yogurt to create a marbled effect.

2. **Serve:** Enjoy this versatile and nutritious dish as a healthy breakfast option or a refreshing snack.

Tips and Variations

- **Protein Boost:** For an extra protein hit, stir in a scoop of your favorite protein powder before adding the toppings.
- **Extra Flavor:** Enhance the flavor by drizzling a little honey or agave syrup over the top if you're not strictly watching your sugar intake.
- **Vegan Option:** Use a plant-based yogurt alternative to make this recipe vegan-friendly.

Storage and Serving Suggestions

- **Freshness:** This dish is best consumed immediately after preparation to enjoy the freshness of the ingredients. If needed, it can be stored in the refrigerator for up to 24 hours.

Nutritional Information per Serving

- **Calories:** Approximately 200-250 kcal (varies by additions)
- **Protein:** High (primarily from Greek yogurt)
- **Carbohydrates:** Moderate (varies depending on the addition of fruits or granola)
- **Fats:** Moderate (from nuts and any added granola)
- **Fiber:** Moderate (from nuts, fruits, and granola)
- **Sodium:** Low

4. OAT AND BANANA PANCAKES

 Prep time: 10 minutes   **Cooking time:** 5 minutes   **Total time:** 15 minutes   **Servings:** 1

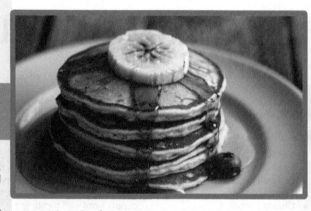

Ingredients

- **Rolled oats:** 1/2 cup (50 g)
- **Banana:** 1 medium, mashed
- **Egg:** 1 large
- **Baking powder:** 1 tsp
- **Vanilla extract:** 1/2 tsp

American Twist:

- **Zero-calorie maple-flavored syrup:** To serve

British Touch:

- **Nutmeg:** 1/4 tsp, grated

Step-by-Step Instructions

1. **Mix Ingredients:** In a blender, combine rolled oats, the mashed banana, egg, baking powder, and vanilla extract.

   - **British Touch:** Add grated nutmeg to the batter for a warm, spicy flavor that complements the sweetness of the banana.
   - **American Twist:** Prepare to serve the pancakes with zero-calorie maple-flavored syrup.

2. **Cook Pancakes:** Heat a non-stick skillet over medium heat and lightly grease it with a bit of oil or butter. Pour small rounds of batter onto the skillet, cooking for about 2 minutes on each side or until golden brown and set.

3. **Serve:** Plate the pancakes. Drizzle with zero-calorie maple-flavored syrup for an American touch, enhancing the pancakes with a sweet, maple flavor without the added calories.

Nutritional Information per Serving

- **Calories:** 350 kcal
- **Protein:** 15 g (30% of RDV)
- **Carbohydrates:** 52 g (18% of RDV)
- **Sugars:** 14 g (no daily recommended value for added sugars)
- **Fat:** 8 g (12% of RDV)
- **Saturated Fat:** 2 g (10% of RDV)
- **Fiber:** 6 g (24% of RDV)
- **Sodium:** 300 mg (13% of RDV)

BREAKFAST

5. CINNAMON OATMEAL PORRIDGE

 Prep time: 5 minutes **Cooking time:** 10 minutes **Total time:** 15 minutes **Servings:** 1

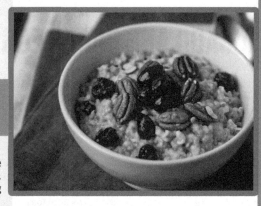

Ingredients
- **Rolled oats:** 1 cup (80 g)
- **Milk:** 2 cups (480 ml)
- **Cinnamon:** 1 tsp
- **Apple:** 1 medium, peeled and diced
- **Salt:** A pinch
- **Optional stevia:** To taste

American Twist:

- **Vanilla extract:** 1/2 tsp
- **Blueberries:** 1/2 cup (75 g)

British Touch:

- **Sultanas:** 1/4 cup (40 g)
- **Single cream:** To serve

Step-by-Step Instructions
1. **Cook Oatmeal:** In a medium saucepan, combine rolled oats, milk, cinnamon, and a pinch of salt. Bring to a simmer over medium heat, stirring frequently to prevent sticking.

2. **Add Apples:** Once the mixture begins to simmer, add the diced apple and continue to cook, stirring occasionally until the oats are soft and the porridge has thickened, about 5-7 minutes.

   - **American Twist:** Stir in vanilla extract with the apples for a rich, aromatic flavor. Serve the cooked oatmeal topped with fresh blueberries, adding a burst of freshness and a touch of American flair.
   - **British Touch:** Add sultanas along with the apples to infuse the porridge with their sweet, distinctive flavor. Serve the porridge with a generous swirl of single cream for a classic British indulgence.

3. **Sweeten and Serve:** Taste the porridge and, if desired, sweeten with stevia. Spoon the hot porridge into a bowl, applying the American or British additions as suggested.

Nutritional Information per Serving
- **Calories:** 350 kcal
- **Protein:** 12 g (24% of RDV)
- **Carbohydrates:** 60 g (22% of RDV)
- **Sugars:** 18 g (no daily recommended value for added sugars)
- **Fat:** 7 g (11% of RDV)
- **Saturated Fat:** 2.5 g (12.5% of RDV)
- **Fiber:** 6 g (24% of RDV)
- **Sodium:** 200 mg (8.7% of RDV)

6. TURKEY AND SPINACH FRITTATA

 Prep time: 10 minutes **Cooking time:** 20 minutes **Total time:** 30 minutes **Servings:** 1

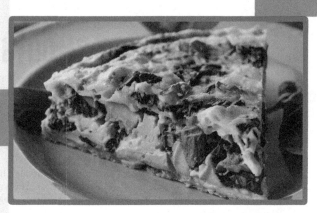

Ingredients
- **Eggs:** 6 large
- **Lean ground turkey:** 1/2 pound (225 g)
- **Fresh spinach:** 1 cup, chopped
- **Tomatoes:** 2 medium, diced
- **Onion:** 1 small, chopped
- **Mixed herbs (such as parsley, thyme, basil):** 1 tbsp, chopped
- **Salt:** 1/2 tsp
- **Pepper:** 1/4 tsp

American Twist:
- **Diced avocado:** 1 medium
- **Monterey Jack cheese:** 1/2 cup (50 g), grated

British Touch:
- **Cooked, sliced new potatoes:** 1/2 cup (100 g)
- **Stilton cheese:** 1/4 cup (30 g), crumbled

Step-by-Step Instructions
1. **Preheat and Prepare:** Preheat the oven to 375°F (190°C). Lightly grease a medium oven-safe skillet or baking dish.

2. **Cook Turkey and Vegetables:** In a large skillet over medium heat, cook the ground turkey until browned. Add the chopped onions, tomatoes, and spinach, cooking until the vegetables are soft and the spinach has wilted, about 5-7 minutes. Season with mixed herbs, salt, and pepper.

3. **Add Eggs:** In a bowl, whisk the eggs until well beaten. Pour the eggs over the cooked turkey and vegetable mixture in the skillet, making sure the eggs are evenly distributed.

   - **American Twist:** Stir in the diced avocado and sprinkle half of the grated Monterey Jack cheese into the egg mixture before it sets.
   - **British Touch:** Layer the cooked, sliced new potatoes on top of the turkey and vegetable mixture, then sprinkle over the crumbled Stilton cheese.

4. **Bake the Frittata:** Transfer the skillet to the preheated oven. Bake for 15-20 minutes or until the eggs are set and the top is lightly golden.

5. **Serve:** Remove the frittata from the oven. If using the American twist, sprinkle the remaining Monterey Jack cheese over the top and let it melt. Slice and serve warm.

Nutritional Information per Serving
- **Calories:** 550 kcal
- **Protein:** 45 g (90% of RDV)
- **Carbohydrates:** 20 g (7% of RDV)
- **Sugars:** 5 g (no daily recommended value for added sugars)
- **Fat:** 35 g (54% of RDV)
- **Saturated Fat:** 12 g (60% of RDV)
- **Fiber:** 5 g (20% of RDV)
- **Sodium:** 800 mg (35% of RDV)

7. AVOCADO AND BAKED EGG TOAST

 Prep time: 5 minutes   **Cooking time:** 15 minutes   **Total time:** 20 minutes **Servings:** 1

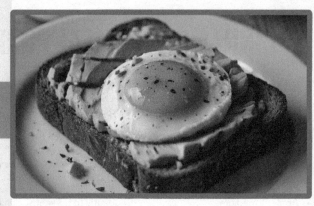

Ingredients
- **Whole grain bread:** 1 slice
- **Avocado:** 1/2, mashed
- **Egg:** 1 large
- **Black pepper:** To taste
- **Salt:** To taste

American Twist:
- **Sriracha or hot sauce:** To drizzle

British Touch:
- **Smoked salmon:** 1 slice
- **or Anchovies:** 3-4 fillets

Step-by-Step Instructions
1. **Preheat Oven:** Preheat your oven to 425°F (220°C) and lightly grease a small baking dish.

2. **Prepare Avocado Toast:** Toast the slice of whole grain bread until it is golden and crispy. Spread the mashed avocado evenly over the toast. Season with salt and black pepper.

3. **Bake the Egg:** Carefully crack the egg over the mashed avocado, trying to keep the yolk intact. Place the toast in the preheated oven and bake for about 10-15 minutes, or until the egg white is set but the yolk remains slightly runny, depending on your preference.

    - **American Twist:** After removing the toast from the oven, drizzle with sriracha or hot sauce for a spicy kick that complements the creamy avocado.
    - **British Touch:** Before baking, top the avocado with a slice of smoked salmon or a few anchovies. The saltiness of the fish will enhance the flavors and add a British flair to this simple dish.

4. **Serve:** Remove the avocado and baked egg toast from the oven, apply the American or British twist as desired, and serve immediately.

Nutritional Information per Serving
- **Calories:** 350 kcal
- **Protein:** 18 g (36% of RDV)
- **Carbohydrates:** 35 g (13% of RDV)
- **Sugars:** 3 g (no daily recommended value for added sugars)
- **Fat:** 20 g (31% of RDV)
- **Saturated Fat:** 4 g (20% of RDV)
- **Fiber:** 9 g (36% of RDV)
- **Sodium:** 400 mg (17% of RDV)

8. CHIA AND BERRY SMOOTHIE BOWL

 Prep time: 15 minutes (includes time for chia seeds to soak)   **Cooking time:** Not Expected   **Total time:** 15 minutes   **Servings:** 1

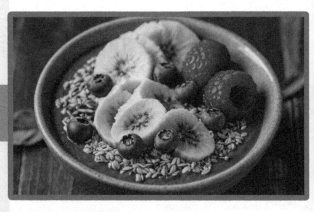

Ingredients
- **Chia seeds:** 3 tbsps
- **Coconut milk:** 1 cup (240 ml)
- **Mixed berries (such as strawberries, blueberries, and raspberries):** 1 cup, fresh or frozen
- **Almonds:** 1/4 cup, sliced or chopped

American Twist:
- **Granola:** 1/4 cup
- **Banana slices:** From 1/2 banana

British Touch:
- **Stewed rhubarb:** 1/4 cup
- **Crushed digestive biscuits:** 2 tbsps

Step-by-Step Instructions
1. **Soak Chia Seeds:** In a medium bowl, combine the chia seeds with coconut milk. Stir well and let sit for about 10 minutes until the mixture begins to thicken.

2. **Prepare Toppings:** While the chia mixture is setting, prepare your choice of toppings based on the desired twist:

    - **American Twist:** Slice half a banana and measure out the granola.
    - **British Touch:** Prepare the stewed rhubarb and crush the digestive biscuits.

3. **Assemble the Smoothie Bowl:** After the chia mixture has thickened, add half of the mixed berries to the bowl and stir gently. Pour the mixture into a serving bowl.

    - **American Twist:** Top the chia and berry mixture with granola, banana slices, and the remaining berries.
    - **British Touch:** Top the chia and berry mixture with stewed rhubarb, crushed digestive biscuits, and the remaining berries.

4. **Serve:** Enjoy your smoothie bowl immediately for the best texture and freshness.

Nutritional Information per Serving
- **Calories:** 480 kcal
- **Protein:** 10 g (20% of RDV)
- **Carbohydrates:** 58 g (21% of RDV)
- **Sugars:** 20 g (no daily recommended value for added sugars)
- **Fat:** 24 g (37% of RDV)
- **Saturated Fat:** 10 g (50% of RDV)
- **Fiber:** 15 g (60% of RDV)
- **Sodium:** 150 mg (6.5% of RDV)

BREAKFAST

9. WHOLE GRAIN APPLE MUFFINS

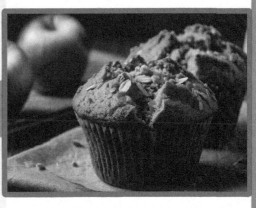

 Prep time: 10 minutes   **Cooking time:** 15-20 minutes 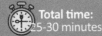 **Total time:** 25-30 minutes **Servings:** 1

Ingredients

- **Whole grain flour:** 1/2 cup (60 g)
- **Apple:** 1 small, peeled and grated
- **Egg:** 1 large
- **Coconut oil:** 2 tbsps (melted)
- **Cinnamon:** 1/4 tsp
- **Baking soda:** 1/4 tsp

American Twist:
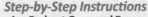
- **Walnuts:** 2 tbsps, chopped
- **Apple cider vinegar:** 1/2 tsp

British Touch:
- **Dried currants:** 2 tbsps
- **Mixed spice:** 1/4 tsp (a blend of cinnamon, nutmeg, and allspice)

Step-by-Step Instructions

1. **Preheat Oven and Prepare Pan:** Preheat your oven to 375°F (190°C). Grease or line a muffin tin with one paper liner for a single serving.

2. **Mix Dry Ingredients:** In a bowl, mix together the whole grain flour, cinnamon, and baking soda.

   - **British Touch:** Add the mixed spice to the dry ingredients for a hint of warm, aromatic flavors.

3. **Combine Wet Ingredients:** In another bowl, whisk together the egg, melted coconut oil, and grated apple.

   - **American Twist:** Stir in the apple cider vinegar to enhance the flavor and help the baking soda react.

4. **Add Ins:** Combine the wet and dry ingredients and stir until just mixed. Avoid overmixing to keep the muffin light and fluffy.

   - **American Twist:** Fold in the chopped walnuts for added texture and nutty flavor.
   - **British Touch:** Mix in the dried currants for bursts of sweetness.

5. **Fill Muffin Cup and Bake:** Spoon the batter into the prepared muffin cup, filling it almost to the top. Place in the preheated oven and bake for 15-20 minutes, or until a toothpick inserted into the center comes out clean.

6. **Cool and Serve:** Allow the muffin to cool in the pan for 5 minutes, then transfer to a wire rack to cool completely. Serve warm or at room temperature.

Nutritional Information per Serving

- **Calories:** 350 kcal
- **Protein:** 8 g (16% of RDV)
- **Carbohydrates:** 45 g (17% of RDV)
- **Sugars:** 12 g (no daily recommended value for added sugars)
- **Fat:** 18 g (28% of RDV)
- **Saturated Fat:** 10 g (50% of RDV)
- **Fiber:** 5 g (20% of RDV)
- **Sodium:** 300 mg (13% of RDV)

10. EGG AND VEGETABLE CASSEROLE

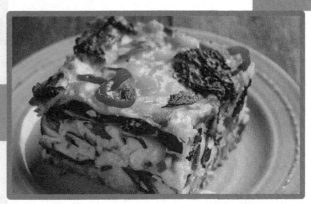

 Prep time: 10 minutes   **Cooking time:** 20 minutes   **Total time:** 30 minutes   **Servings:** 1

Ingredients

- **Eggs:** 2 large
- **Zucchini:** 1/4 medium, sliced
- **Bell peppers:** 1/4 large, diced
- **Onions:** 1/4 small, diced
- **Spinach:** 1/2 cup, chopped
- **Optional low-fat cheese:** 2 tbsps, grated

American Twist:
- **Sweet corn:** 2 tbsps
- **Paprika:** 1/4 tsp

British Touch:

- **Leeks:** 1/4 large, sliced
- **Mustard powder:** 1/4 tsp

Step-by-Step Instructions

1. **Preheat Oven and Prepare Dish:** Preheat your oven to 375°F (190°C). Lightly grease a small baking dish suitable for a single serving.

2. **Sauté Vegetables:** In a skillet over medium heat, sauté the onions, bell peppers, and zucchini until they are soft, about 5 minutes. If using the British touch, also include the leeks in this step.

   - **American Twist:** After the vegetables are sautéed, stir in the sweet corn to mix well with the other vegetables.

3. **Prepare Egg Mixture:** In a bowl, whisk the eggs with salt and pepper.

   - **American Twist:** Add paprika to the egg mixture for a smoky flavor.
   - **British Touch:** Whisk mustard powder into the egg mixture to infuse it with a distinct pungent flavor.

4. **Combine and Assemble:** Spread the sautéed vegetables evenly in the prepared baking dish. Pour the egg mixture over the vegetables. If using, sprinkle the grated low-fat cheese evenly on top.

5. **Bake:** Place the dish in the preheated oven and bake for about 15-20 minutes, or until the eggs are set and the top is lightly golden.

6. **Serve:** Remove from the oven, let cool slightly, and serve warm.

Nutritional Information per Serving

- **Calories:** 280 kcal
- **Protein:** 20 g (40% of RDV)
- **Carbohydrates:** 18 g (7% of RDV)
- **Sugars:** 8 g (no daily recommended value for added sugars)
- **Fat:** 15 g (23% of RDV)
- **Saturated Fat:** 5 g (25% of RDV)
- **Fiber:** 3 g (12% of RDV)
- **Sodium:** 320 mg (14% of RDV)

11. OAT AND BANANA BARS

 Prep time: 10 minutes   **Cooking time:** 20 minutes   **Total time:** 30 minutes **Servings:** 1

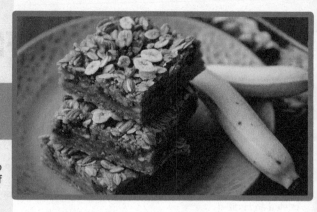

Ingredients
- **Rolled oats:** 1 cup (80 g)
- **Banana:** 1 medium, mashed
- **Egg:** 1
- **Honey:** 2 tbsps (30 ml)
- **Cinnamon:** 1/2 tsp

American Twist:
- **Chocolate chips:** 2 tbsps
- **Sea salt:** a pinch (to sprinkle on top)

British Touch:
- **Sultanas:** 2 tbsps
- **Nutmeg:** 1/4 tsp

Step-by-Step Instructions
1. **Preheat Oven and Prepare Pan:** Preheat your oven to 350°F (175°C). Line a small baking tray or use a mini loaf pan with parchment paper.

2. **Mix Ingredients:** In a large bowl, combine the rolled oats, mashed banana, egg, honey, and cinnamon. Mix thoroughly to form a homogeneous batter.

   - **British Touch:** Stir in the sultanas and nutmeg into the batter to integrate these flavors throughout the bars.
   - **Add American Twist:** Fold in the chocolate chips into the batter. This will give the bars a rich, chocolatey taste and a delightful texture contrast.

3. **Prepare to Bake:** Transfer the mixture into the prepared baking tray or mini loaf pan. Smooth the top with the back of a spoon.

   - **American Twist:** Sprinkle a pinch of sea salt over the top of the mixture before baking, enhancing the sweet flavors with a touch of saltiness.

4. **Bake:** Place the tray in the preheated oven and bake for about 20 minutes, or until the edges are golden brown and a toothpick inserted into the center comes out clean.

5. **Cool and Serve:** Allow the bar to cool in the pan for about 10 minutes, then transfer to a wire rack to cool completely. Slice if necessary and enjoy as a hearty snack or a quick breakfast.

Nutritional Information per Serving
- **Calories:** 480 kcal
- **Protein:** 12 g (24% of RDV)
- **Carbohydrates:** 68 g (26% of RDV)
- **Sugars:** 28 g (no daily recommended value for added sugars)
- **Fat:** 18 g (28% of RDV)
- **Saturated Fat:** 6 g (30% of RDV)
- **Fiber:** 8 g (32% of RDV)
- **Sodium:** 120 mg (5% of RDV)

12. RICOTTA AND FRUIT CREAM WITH NUTS

 Prep time: 5 minutes   **Cooking time:** Not Expected   **Total time:** 5 minutes **Servings:** 1

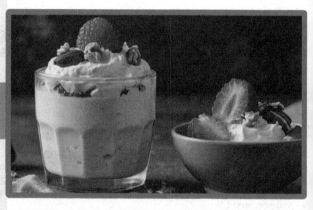

Ingredients
- **Low-fat ricotta:** 1/2 cup (125 g)
- **Fresh fruit (such as strawberries and blueberries):** 1/2 cup (75 g)
- **Chopped nuts (such as almonds or walnuts):** 2 tbsps (15 g)
- **Honey:** 1 tbsp (15 ml)

American Twist:
- **Toasted pecans:** 1 tbsp, chopped
- **Maple syrup:** 1 tsp

British Touch:
- **Mixed berries (additional to the main fruits, such as raspberries or blackberries):** 1/4 cup (37 g)
- **Elderflower cordial:** 1 tsp

Step-by-Step Instructions
1. **Prepare the Ricotta Mix:** In a mixing bowl, combine the ricotta and honey until smooth.

   - **British Touch:** Stir in the elderflower cordial with the ricotta mix to add a subtle floral flavor that complements the sweetness of the fruits.

2. **Prepare the Fruits and Nuts:** Wash and prepare the strawberries, blueberries, and any additional berries. Chop the nuts if they aren't already prepped.

   - **American Twist:** Add toasted pecans to the mix for a nutty flavor and a crunchy texture.

3. **Assemble the Dish:** Spoon the ricotta mix into a serving bowl. Top with the prepared fresh fruits and chopped nuts.

   - **American Twist:** Drizzle maple syrup over the top for a rich, sweet finish.
   - **British Touch:** Add the mixed berries on top of the ricotta to enhance the flavors with more variety and color.

4. **Serve:** Enjoy your creamy and refreshing bowl immediately for the best taste and texture.

Nutritional Information per Serving
- **Calories:** 295 kcal
- **Protein:** 14 g (28% of RDV)
- **Carbohydrates:** 32 g (12% of RDV)
- **Sugars:** 22 g (no daily recommended value for added sugars)
- **Fat:** 13 g (20% of RDV)
- **Saturated Fat:** 5 g (25% of RDV)
- **Fiber:** 4 g (16% of RDV)
- **Sodium:** 125 mg (5% of RDV)

BREAKFAST

13. CHICKEN CAESAR SALAD

 Prep time: 10 minutes   **Cooking time:** Not Expected   **Total time:** 10 minutes   **Servings:** 1

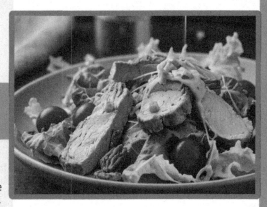

Ingredients
- **Grilled chicken breast:** 1 large, sliced
- **Romaine lettuce:** 2 cups, chopped
- **Cherry tomatoes:** 1/2 cup, halved
- **Parmesan shavings:** 1/4 cup

American Twist:
- **Croutons:** 1/2 cup

British Touch:
- **Watercress:** 2 cups (replace romaine lettuce)

Step-by-Step Instructions
1. **Prepare the Base Salad:**

   • If opting for the traditional American style, place the chopped romaine lettuce in a large salad bowl.
   • For the British twist, substitute the romaine with fresh watercress to add a peppery flavor to the salad.

2. **Add Chicken and Tomatoes:** Arrange the sliced grilled chicken and halved cherry tomatoes over the lettuce or watercress.

3. **Add Parmesan:** Sprinkle the parmesan shavings generously over the top of the salad.

   • **American Twist:** Add croutons to the salad for a satisfying crunch and a traditional Caesar salad experience.

4. **Dressing:** Drizzle your favorite Caesar dressing over the salad. Toss all the ingredients lightly to combine and coat evenly with the dressing.

5. **Serve:** Serve the salad immediately after dressing to maintain the freshness and crunch of the greens and croutons.

Nutritional Information per Serving
- **Calories:** 450 kcal
- **Protein:** 38 g (76% of RDV)
- **Carbohydrates:** 12 g (4% of RDV)
- **Sugars:** 3 g (no daily recommended value for added sugars)
- **Fat:** 28 g (43% of RDV)
- **Saturated Fat:** 8 g (40% of RDV)
- **Fiber:** 3 g (12% of RDV)
- **Sodium:** 580 mg (25% of RDV)

14. TURKEY AND AVOCADO SALAD

 Prep time: 10 minutes   **Cooking time:** Not Expected   **Total time:** 10 minutes   **Servings:** 1

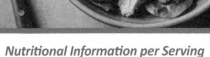

Ingredients
- **Smoked turkey breast:** 1 cup, sliced
- **Avocado:** 1 medium, sliced
- **Mixed greens:** 2 cups
- **Red onion:** 1/4 cup, thinly sliced

American Twist:
- **Crispy bacon:** 2 slices, cooked and crumbled

British Touch:
- **Sliced radishes:** 1/4 cup

Step-by-Step Instructions
1. **Prepare the Ingredients:** Wash and dry the mixed greens. Peel and slice the avocado, and thinly slice the red onion. If using radishes for the British touch, slice them thinly.

2. **Assemble the Salad:** In a large bowl, combine the mixed greens, sliced smoked turkey, avocado, and red onion.

   • **American Twist:** Add the crumbled crispy bacon to the salad for a savory crunch that complements the creamy avocado and smoked turkey.
   • **British Touch:** Include the sliced radishes for a crisp, peppery contrast that enhances the overall freshness of the salad.

3. **Dressing:** Drizzle your choice of dressing over the salad. A light vinaigrette or a creamy avocado dressing works well with this mix.

4. **Toss and Serve:** Gently toss the salad to evenly distribute the dressing and ingredients. Serve immediately to maintain the freshness and textures of the ingredients.

Nutritional Information per Serving
- **Calories:** 370 kcal
- **Protein:** 25 g (50% of RDV)
- **Carbohydrates:** 15 g (5% of RDV)
- **Sugars:** 3 g (no daily recommended value for added sugars)
- **Fat:** 25 g (38% of RDV)
- **Saturated Fat:** 5 g (25% of RDV)
- **Fiber:** 7 g (28% of RDV)
- **Sodium:** 350 mg (15% of RDV)

15. EGG AND SPINACH SALAD

 Prep time: 10 minutes   **Cooking time:** Not Expected **Total time:** 10 minutes **Servings:** 1

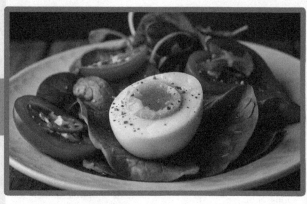

Ingredients

- **Hard-boiled eggs:** 2, peeled and quartered
- **Fresh spinach:** 1 cup
- **Bell peppers:** 1/4 cup, thinly sliced
- **Cucumber:** 1/4 cup, sliced

American Twist:
- **Ranch dressing:** 2 tbsps

British Touch:
- **Mustard vinaigrette:** 2 tbsps (prepare by mixing 1 tbsp olive oil, 1/2 tbsp vinegar, 1/2 tsp mustard, salt, and pepper)

Step-by-Step Instructions

1. **Prepare Ingredients:** Begin by washing and drying the fresh spinach. Slice the bell peppers and cucumber, and quarter the hard-boiled eggs.

2. **Assemble the Salad:** In a large bowl, combine the spinach, bell peppers, cucumber, and eggs. Toss lightly to mix the ingredients.

   - **American Twist:** Drizzle ranch dressing over the salad and toss well to coat each ingredient thoroughly. The creamy richness of the ranch dressing adds a comforting and familiar American flavor to the salad.
   - **British Touch:** Pour the mustard vinaigrette over the salad and toss to combine. The sharpness of the mustard vinaigrette complements the fresh vegetables and eggs, lending a distinctly British flavor to the dish.

3. **Serve:** Plate the salad immediately after dressing to maintain the freshness and crispness of the vegetables.

Nutritional Information per Serving
- **Calories:** 350 kcal
- **Protein:** 14 g (28% of RDV)
- **Carbohydrates:** 12 g (4% of RDV)
- **Sugars:** 4 g (no daily recommended value for added sugars)
- **Fat:** 27 g (42% of RDV)
- **Saturated Fat:** 6 g (30% of RDV)
- **Fiber:** 3 g (12% of RDV)
- **Sodium:** 300 mg (13% of RDV)

16. CHICKPEA AND QUINOA SALAD

 Prep time: 10 minutes   **Cooking time:** Not Expected   **Total time:** 10 minutes   **Servings:** 1

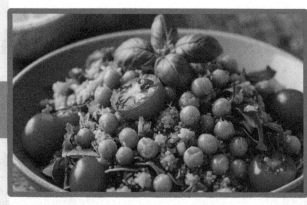

Ingredients

- **Cooked quinoa:** 1/2 cup
- **Chickpeas:** 1/2 cup, drained and rinsed
- **Cherry tomatoes:** 1/4 cup, halved
- **Parsley:** 2 tbsps, chopped
- **Lemon dressing:** 1 tbsp (mix 2 tsps olive oil, 1 tsp lemon juice, salt, and pepper to taste)

American Twist:
- **Feta cheese:** 2 tbsps, crumbled

British Touch:
- **Roasted beetroot:** 1/4 cup, diced

Step-by-Step Instructions

1. **Prepare Ingredients:** Cook the quinoa according to package instructions if not already prepared. Allow it to cool. Meanwhile, prepare the cherry tomatoes, parsley, and if using, the roasted beetroot.

2. **Assemble the Salad:** In a mixing bowl, combine the cooked quinoa, chickpeas, cherry tomatoes, and chopped parsley.

   - **British Touch:** Add the roasted beetroot to the salad for a sweet, earthy flavor that pairs beautifully with the nutty quinoa and chickpeas.

3. **Add Dressing:** Drizzle the lemon dressing over the salad and toss well to ensure all ingredients are evenly coated.

   - **American Twist:** Sprinkle the crumbled feta cheese over the salad after dressing. The salty creaminess of the feta adds a rich depth to the light and refreshing ingredients.

4. **Serve:** Mix thoroughly once more before serving to blend all flavors. Enjoy this nutritious salad as a vibrant lunch or a healthy side dish.

Nutritional Information per Serving
- **Calories:** 370 kcal
- **Protein:** 14 g (28% of RDV)
- **Carbohydrates:** 45 g (17% of RDV)
- **Sugars:** 7 g (no daily recommended value for added sugars)
- **Fat:** 15 g (23% of RDV)
- **Saturated Fat:** 3 g (15% of RDV)
- **Fiber:** 8 g (32% of RDV)
- **Sodium:** 300 mg (13% of RDV)

17. CHICKEN VEGETABLE SOUP

 Prep time: 10 minutes   **Cooking time:** 30 minutes   **Total time:** 40 minutes   **Servings:** 1

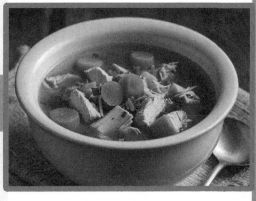

Ingredients
- **Diced chicken breast:** 1/2 cup (about 100 g)
- **Carrots:** 1/4 cup, diced
- **Celery:** 1/4 cup, diced
- **Onions:** 1/4 cup, diced
- **Chicken broth:** 2 cups (480 ml)

American Twist:
- **Noodles:** 1/4 cup, uncooked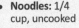

British Touch:
- **Pearl barley:** 2 tbsps, rinsed

Step-by-Step Instructions
1. **Prepare Ingredients:** Dice the chicken breast, carrots, celery, and onions. If using pearl barley, rinse it thoroughly under cold water.

2. **Cook the Soup:** In a medium saucepan, combine the diced chicken, carrots, celery, onions, and chicken broth. Bring the mixture to a boil over medium heat.

   • **British Touch:** Add the rinsed pearl barley to the saucepan at the beginning of cooking. Pearl barley will take about 25-30 minutes to cook, making it tender and adding a nutty flavor and hearty texture to the soup.

3. **Simmer:** Reduce the heat to low and let the soup simmer gently. If you are not using pearl barley, let it simmer for about 20 minutes, or until the vegetables and chicken are tender.

   • **American Twist:** Add the uncooked noodles to the soup about 10 minutes before the end of cooking. This will give the noodles enough time to cook through and absorb the flavors of the broth.

4. **Adjust Seasonings:** After the soup has finished cooking, taste and adjust the seasonings, adding salt and pepper as needed.

5. **Serve:** Ladle the hot soup into a bowl. If you've added noodles, ensure they're evenly distributed in the serving.

Nutritional Information per Serving
- **Calories:** 320 kcal
- **Protein:** 28 g (56% of RDV)
- **Carbohydrates:** 28 g (11% of RDV)
- **Sugars:** 5 g (no daily recommended value for added sugars)
- **Fat:** 8 g (12% of RDV)
- **Saturated Fat:** 2 g (10% of RDV)
- **Fiber:** 4 g (16% of RDV)
- **Sodium:** 800 mg (35% of RDV)

18. BEEF AND VEGETABLE BROTH

 Prep time: 10 minutes   **Cooking time:** 35 minutes   **Total time:** 45 minutes   **Servings:** 1

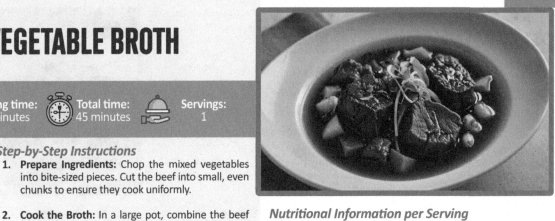

Ingredients
- **Lean beef chunks:** 1/2 cup (about 100 g)
- **Mixed vegetables (such as carrots, celery, and peas):** 1 cup
- **Beef broth:** 2 cups (480 ml)
- **Herbs (such as thyme and parsley):** 1 tsp, chopped

American Twist:
- **Cornbread:** 1 slice, to serve

British Touch:
- **Worcestershire sauce:** 1 tbsp

Step-by-Step Instructions
1. **Prepare Ingredients:** Chop the mixed vegetables into bite-sized pieces. Cut the beef into small, even chunks to ensure they cook uniformly.

2. **Cook the Broth:** In a large pot, combine the beef chunks, mixed vegetables, beef broth, and herbs. Bring the mixture to a boil over medium-high heat.

   • **British Touch:** Add Worcestershire sauce to the pot at the beginning of cooking. This will infuse the broth with a deep, savory flavor, enhancing the richness of the beef.

3. **Simmer:** Once boiling, reduce the heat to a simmer. Let the broth cook uncovered for about 30-35 minutes, or until the beef is tender and the vegetables are cooked through.

4. **Adjust Seasonings:** Taste the broth and adjust the seasonings with salt and pepper as needed.

5. **Serve:** Ladle the hot broth into a bowl.

   • **American Twist:** Serve with a warm slice of cornbread on the side for a comforting American-style meal.

Nutritional Information per Serving
- **Calories:** 300 kcal
- **Protein:** 25 g (50% of RDV)
- **Carbohydrates:** 20 g (8% of RDV)
- **Sugars:** 5 g (no daily recommended value for added sugars)
- **Fat:** 10 g (15% of RDV)
- **Saturated Fat:** 3 g (15% of RDV)
- **Fiber:** 4 g (16% of RDV)
- **Sodium:** 950 mg (42% of RDV)

19. LENTIL TOMATO SOUP

 Prep time: 5 minutes   **Cooking time:** 25 minutes   **Total time:** 30 minutes   **Servings:** 1

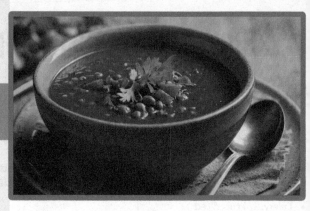

Ingredients

- **Red lentils:** 1/2 cup (100 g), rinsed
- **Tomato puree:** 1 cup (240 ml)
- **Carrots:** 1/4 cup, diced
- **Celery:** 1/4 cup, diced
- **Vegetable broth:** 2 cups (480 ml)

American Twist:
- **Smoked paprika:** 1/2 tsp

British Touch:
- **Fresh thyme:** 1 tsp, finely chopped

Step-by-Step Instructions

1. **Prepare the Ingredients:** Dice the carrots and celery into small, even pieces. Rinse the red lentils under cold water until the water runs clear.

2. **Cook the Soup:** In a medium pot, combine the red lentils, tomato puree, diced carrots, celery, and vegetable broth. Bring the mixture to a boil over medium heat.

    - **British Touch:** Add fresh thyme to the pot. The herb will infuse the soup with a subtle, earthy flavor that complements the richness of the tomatoes and the heartiness of the lentils.

3. **Simmer:** Once boiling, reduce the heat to low, cover, and let the soup simmer gently for about 20 minutes, or until the lentils and vegetables are soft.

    - **American Twist:** Stir in smoked paprika halfway through the simmering process. This will add a warm, smoky depth to the soup, enhancing its overall flavor profile.

4. **Blend (Optional):** For a smoother texture, use an immersion blender to partially or fully puree the soup, depending on your preference.

5. **Season and Serve:** Adjust the seasoning with salt and pepper to taste. Serve the soup hot, with a crusty piece of bread if desired.

Nutritional Information per Serving
- **Calories:** 280 kcal
- **Protein:** 18 g (36% of RDV)
- **Carbohydrates:** 40 g (15% of RDV)
- **Sugars:** 8 g (no daily recommended value for added sugars)
- **Fat:** 2 g (3% of RDV)
- **Saturated Fat:** 0 g (0% of RDV)
- **Fiber:** 10 g (40% of RDV)
- **Sodium:** 600 mg (26% of RDV)

20. SEAFOOD CHOWDER

 Prep time: 10 minutes   **Cooking time:** 30 minutes   **Total time:** 40 minutes   **Servings:** 1

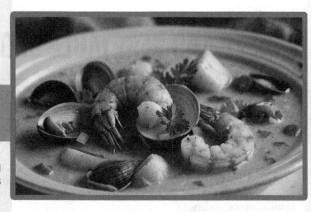

Ingredients

- **Mixed seafood (such as shrimp, scallops, and clams):** 1 cup
- **Potatoes:** 1/2 cup, diced
- **Onions:** 1/4 cup, finely chopped
- **Fish broth:** 2 cups (480 ml)
- **Light cream:** 1/2 cup (120 ml)

American Twist:
- **Sweet corn:** 1/4 cup

British Touch:
- **Saffron:** A pinch

Step-by-Step Instructions

1. **Prepare Ingredients:** Peel and dice the potatoes, and finely chop the onions. If using frozen seafood, ensure it's thawed and drained.

2. **Cook the Base:** In a large pot, sauté the onions over medium heat until translucent. Add the diced potatoes and fish broth, bringing the mixture to a simmer.

3. **Add Seafood:** Once the potatoes are nearly tender, add the mixed seafood to the pot. Simmer gently to avoid overcooking the seafood, which should take about 5-7 minutes until everything is cooked through.

    - **British Touch:** Add a pinch of saffron when you add the seafood. Saffron will infuse the chowder with a beautiful color and a rich, aromatic flavor, enhancing the depth of the dish.

4. **Add Cream and Final Touches:** Reduce the heat to low and stir in the light cream, heating through without bringing it to a boil to prevent curdling.

    - **American Twist:** Stir in the sweet corn along with the light cream for a pop of sweetness and color, contributing to the classic American chowder profile.

5. **Season and Serve:** Season the chowder with salt and pepper to taste. Serve hot, garnished with a sprinkle of chopped parsley or chives for added freshness.

Nutritional Information per Serving
- **Calories:** 450 kcal
- **Protein:** 25 g (50% of RDV)
- **Carbohydrates:** 38 g (14% of RDV)
- **Sugars:** 5 g (no daily recommended value for added sugars)
- **Fat:** 20 g (31% of RDV)
- **Saturated Fat:** 10 g (50% of RDV)
- **Fiber:** 4 g (16% of RDV)
- **Sodium:** 950 mg (41% of RDV)

21. CHICKEN STIR-FRY

 Prep time: 10 minutes **Cooking time:** 15 minutes **Total time:** 25 minutes **Servings:** 1

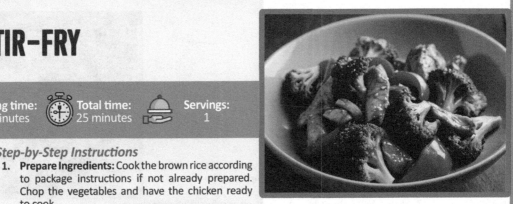

Ingredients

- **Diced chicken breast:** 1/2 cup (about 100 g)
- **Broccoli:** 1/2 cup, cut into florets
- **Bell peppers:** 1/4 cup, sliced
- **Soy sauce:** 1 tbsp (use hoisin sauce for the British touch)
- **Brown rice:** 1/2 cup, cooked

American Twist:
- **Peanut sauce:** 2 tbsps, to serve

British Touch:
- **Hoisin sauce:** Replace soy sauce with 1 tbsp hoisin sauce

Step-by-Step Instructions

1. **Prepare Ingredients:** Cook the brown rice according to package instructions if not already prepared. Chop the vegetables and have the chicken ready to cook.

2. **Cook Chicken:** In a large skillet or wok, heat a little oil over medium-high heat. Add the diced chicken breast and stir-fry until it is nearly cooked through, about 5-7 minutes.

3. **Add Vegetables:** Add the broccoli and bell peppers to the skillet. Stir-fry the vegetables with the chicken until they are tender but still crisp, about 3-4 minutes.

   • **British Touch:** Instead of soy sauce, use hoisin sauce for a richer, slightly sweeter flavor that complements the stir-fry well.

4. **Season:** Pour the soy sauce (or hoisin sauce) over the chicken and vegetables. Stir well to ensure everything is evenly coated and cook for an additional minute.

5. **Serve:** Spoon the stir-fry over the cooked brown rice.

   • **American Twist:** Serve the stir-fry with peanut sauce on the side, allowing for a creamy, rich addition that enhances the dish with a distinctly American flavor.

6. **Enjoy:** Serve hot, garnished with sesame seeds or green onions if desired.

Nutritional Information per Serving
- **Calories:** 420 kcal
- **Protein:** 30 g (60% of RDV)
- **Carbohydrates:** 45 g (17% of RDV)
- **Sugars:** 5 g (no daily recommended value for added sugars)
- **Fat:** 15 g (23% of RDV)
- **Saturated Fat:** 3 g (15% of RDV)
- **Fiber:** 5 g (20% of RDV)
- **Sodium:** 950 mg (41% of RDV)

22. TURKEY CASSEROLE

 Prep time: 15 minutes **Cooking time:** 25 minutes **Total time:** 40 minutes **Servings:** 1

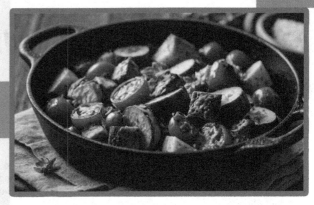

Ingredients

- **Ground turkey:** 1/2 cup (about 100 g)
- **Diced tomatoes:** 1/2 cup (canned or fresh)
- **Zucchini:** 1/4 cup, diced
- **Onions:** 1/4 cup, diced
- **Herbs (such as basil, oregano, or thyme):** 1 tsp, mixed and chopped

American Twist:
- **Low-fat cheese:** 1/4 cup, shredded

British Touch:
- **Mashed cauliflower:** 1/2 cup, prepared

Step-by-Step Instructions

1. **Preheat Oven and Prepare Ingredients:** Preheat your oven to 375°F (190°C). Dice the zucchini and onions, and prepare the mashed cauliflower if using the British touch.

2. **Cook Turkey and Vegetables:** In a medium skillet over medium heat, cook the ground turkey until it's no longer pink, about 5-7 minutes. Add the onions and zucchini, cooking until they are softened, about 5 minutes. Stir in the diced tomatoes and herbs, and let simmer for another 5 minutes until everything is well combined.

3. **Assemble the Casserole:** Transfer the turkey and vegetable mixture to a small baking dish suitable for one serving.

   • **American Twist:** Sprinkle shredded low-fat cheese over the top of the turkey mixture. The cheese will melt and brown in the oven, adding a deliciously gooey texture and rich flavor.
   • **British Touch:** Instead of cheese, cover the turkey mixture with a layer of mashed cauliflower. This creates a low-carb crust that will brown nicely in the oven, providing a satisfying contrast in textures.

4. **Bake:** Place the casserole in the preheated oven and bake for 15-20 minutes, or until the topping is golden and the casserole is heated through.

5. **Serve:** Remove the casserole from the oven and let it sit for a few minutes before serving. This allows the flavors to meld together beautifully.

Nutritional Information per Serving
- **Calories:** 350 kcal
- **Protein:** 28 g (56% of RDV)
- **Carbohydrates:** 15 g (6% of RDV)
- **Sugars:** 8 g (no daily recommended value for added sugars)
- **Fat:** 18 g (28% of RDV)
- **Saturated Fat:** 5 g (25% of RDV)
- **Fiber:** 3 g (12% of RDV)
- **Sodium:** 300 mg (13% of RDV)

23. VEGETABLE FRITTATA

 Prep time: 10 minutes   **Cooking time:** 20 minutes   **Total time:** 30 minutes   **Servings:** 1

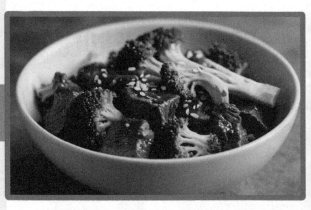

Ingredients

- **Eggs:** 3 large
- **Spinach:** 1/2 cup, chopped
- **Tomatoes:** 1/4 cup, diced
- **Onions:** 1/4 cup, diced
- **Low-fat cheese:** 1/4 cup, grated

American Twist:

- **Diced potatoes:** 1/4 cup, pre-cooked

British Touch:

- **Leeks:** 1/4 cup, finely sliced
- **Cheddar cheese:** 1/4 cup, grated (replace low-fat cheese)

Step-by-Step Instructions

1. **Preheat Oven:** Preheat your oven to 375°F (190°C), ensuring it's hot and ready for the frittata.

2. **Sauté Vegetables:** In a medium oven-safe skillet over medium heat, sauté the onions (and leeks if using the British touch) until they're soft and translucent, about 5 minutes. Add the chopped spinach and cook until wilted, about 2 minutes. If using the American twist, add the diced potatoes to the skillet at this stage and cook until they are lightly browned.

3. **Add Eggs and Cheese:** In a bowl, beat the eggs and pour them over the sautéed vegetables in the skillet. Allow the eggs to set slightly on the bottom, then sprinkle with low-fat cheese or cheddar if following the British touch.

4. **Bake the Frittata:** Transfer the skillet to the preheated oven. Bake for about 10-15 minutes, or until the eggs are fully set and the top of the frittata is lightly golden.

5. **Serve:** Remove the frittata from the oven, let it cool for a few minutes, then slice and serve hot. The frittata should be fluffy and evenly cooked through, with the cheese melted and slightly browned on top.

Nutritional Information per Serving

- **Calories:** 400 kcal
- **Protein:** 28 g (56% of RDV)
- **Carbohydrates:** 20 g (8% of RDV)
- **Sugars:** 5 g (no daily recommended value for added sugars)
- **Fat:** 25 g (38% of RDV)
- **Saturated Fat:** 10 g (50% of RDV)
- **Fiber:** 3 g (12% of RDV)
- **Sodium:** 450 mg (19% of RDV)

24. BEEF AND BROCCOLI BOWL

 Prep time: 10 minutes   **Cooking time:** 15 minutes   **Total time:** 25 minutes   **Servings:** 1

Ingredients

- **Sliced lean beef:** 1/2 cup (about 100 g)
- **Broccoli:** 1/2 cup, cut into florets
- **Garlic:** 1 clove, minced
- **Soy sauce:** 1 tbsp
- **Ginger:** 1 tsp, grated

American Twist: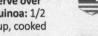

- **Serve over quinoa:** 1/2 cup, cooked

British Touch:

- **Accompany with mashed turnips:** 1/2 cup, cooked and mashed

Step-by-Step Instructions

1. **Prepare Ingredients:** Cook the quinoa according to package instructions if following the American twist. For the British touch, peel, boil, and mash the turnips.

2. **Cook Broccoli:** Steam or blanch the broccoli florets until they are bright green and just tender, about 3-4 minutes. Set aside.

3. **Cook Beef:** In a skillet over medium-high heat, add a little oil. Sauté the minced garlic and grated ginger for about 1 minute until fragrant. Add the sliced beef and stir-fry until browned and nearly cooked through, about 3-5 minutes.

4. **Combine and Sauce:** Add the cooked broccoli to the skillet with the beef. Pour over the soy sauce and toss everything together to coat the beef and broccoli in the sauce. Cook for an additional 2 minutes to allow flavors to meld.

5. **Serve:**

   - **American Twist:** Spoon the beef and broccoli over the cooked quinoa, creating a hearty and nutritious bowl.

   - **British Touch:** Serve the beef and broccoli alongside the mashed turnips for a comforting and traditional British meal.

Nutritional Information per Serving

- **Calories:** 320 kcal
- **Protein:** 28 g (56% of RDV)
- **Carbohydrates:** 25 g (10% of RDV)
- **Sugars:** 3 g (no daily recommended value for added sugars)
- **Fat:** 10 g (15% of RDV)
- **Saturated Fat:** 3 g (15% of RDV)
- **Fiber:** 5 g (20% of RDV)
- **Sodium:** 800 mg (35% of RDV)

25. CHICKEN SALAD WRAP

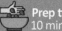 **Prep time:** 10 minutes   **Cooking time:** Not Expected   **Total time:** 10 minutes  **Servings:** 1

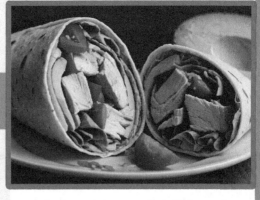

Ingredients

- **Diced chicken:** 1/2 cup (cooked and cooled)
- **Celery:** 1/4 cup, finely chopped
- **Low-fat mayonnaise:** 2 tbsps
- **Whole wheat wrap:** 1

American Twist:
- **Avocado:** 1/4, sliced

British Touch:
- **Watercress:** 1/4 cup

Step-by-Step Instructions

1. **Make Chicken Salad:** In a bowl, combine the diced chicken, chopped celery, and low-fat mayonnaise. Mix thoroughly until all ingredients are well-coated with mayonnaise.

2. **Prepare the Wrap:** Lay the whole wheat wrap flat on a clean surface.

3. **Add Fillings:**
   - **Base Layer:** Spoon the chicken salad onto the center of the wrap, spreading it evenly but leaving enough space at the edges for folding.
   - **American Twist:** Add slices of avocado on top of the chicken salad. The creamy texture of the avocado adds richness and a subtle nutty flavor that complements the chicken.
   - **British Touch:** Add a layer of watercress over the chicken salad. Watercress offers a peppery bite, which contrasts nicely with the creamy chicken salad and adds a burst of color.

4. **Wrap It Up:** Fold the bottom of the wrap up over the fillings, then fold in the sides. Roll the wrap tightly towards the top edge to secure the fillings.

5. **Serve:** Cut the wrap in half diagonally to make it easier to eat. Serve immediately, or wrap in foil to take on the go.

Nutritional Information per Serving
- **Calories:** 350 kcal
- **Protein:** 25 g (50% of RDV)
- **Carbohydrates:** 30 g (12% of RDV)
- **Sugars:** 2 g (no daily recommended value for added sugars)
- **Fat:** 15 g (23% of RDV)
- **Saturated Fat:** 2.5 g (12.5% of RDV)
- **Fiber:** 5 g (20% of RDV)
- **Sodium:** 600 mg (26% of RDV)

26. TUNA SALAD SANDWICH

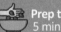 **Prep time:** 5 minutes   **Cooking time:** Not Expected   **Total time:** 5 minutes   **Servings:** 1

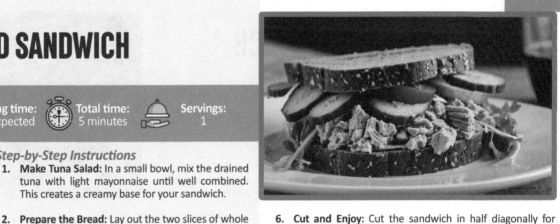

Ingredients

- **Canned tuna:** 1/2 cup, drained
- **Light mayonnaise:** 2 tbsps
- **Cucumber:** 1/4 cup, thinly sliced
- **Whole grain bread:** 2 slices

American Twist:
- **Sliced pickles:** 1/4 cup

British Touch:
- **Cress:** 1/4 cup

Step-by-Step Instructions

1. **Make Tuna Salad:** In a small bowl, mix the drained tuna with light mayonnaise until well combined. This creates a creamy base for your sandwich.

2. **Prepare the Bread:** Lay out the two slices of whole grain bread on a clean surface.

3. **Assemble the Sandwich:** Spread the tuna salad evenly over one slice of bread.

4. **Add Cucumber:** Layer the thinly sliced cucumber over the tuna salad.
   - **American Twist:** Add sliced pickles on top of the cucumber for a tangy crunch that enhances the flavor of the tuna.
   - **British Touch:** Instead of pickles, sprinkle cress over the cucumber. The cress adds a peppery zest that complements the creamy texture of the tuna salad.

5. **Top and Serve:** Place the second slice of bread on top to complete the sandwich. Press down lightly to ensure everything holds together.

6. **Cut and Enjoy:** Cut the sandwich in half diagonally for easier eating. Serve immediately, or wrap for a convenient on-the-go meal.

Nutritional Information per Serving
- **Calories:** 320 kcal
- **Protein:** 25 g (50% of RDV)
- **Carbohydrates:** 35 g (14% of RDV)
- **Sugars:** 4 g (no daily recommended value for added sugars)
- **Fat:** 10 g (15% of RDV)
- **Saturated Fat:** 2 g (10% of RDV)
- **Fiber:** 5 g (20% of RDV)
- **Sodium:** 720 mg (31% of RDV)

27. TURKEY AND CRANBERRY WRAP

 Prep time: 5 minutes   **Cooking time:** Not Expected   **Total time:** 5 minutes   **Servings:** 1

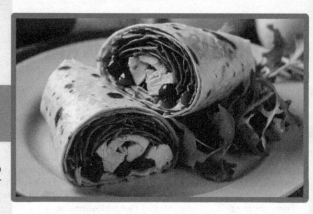

Ingredients

- **Sliced turkey:** 1/2 cup
- **Cranberry sauce:** 2 tbsps
- **Spinach:** 1/2 cup (substitute with rocket for the British touch)
- **Whole wheat wrap:** 1

American Twist:

- **Cream cheese:** 2 tbsps

British Touch:

- **Use rocket (arugula):** 1/2 cup instead of spinach

Step-by-Step Instructions

1. **Prepare the Wrap:** Lay the whole wheat wrap flat on a clean surface. This acts as your base for building the wrap.

2. **Spread Condiments:**
   - **American Twist:** Spread cream cheese evenly over the surface of the wrap before adding other ingredients. The cream cheese adds a rich, smooth texture that pairs wonderfully with the tart cranberry sauce.
   - If using the **British touch**, prepare the rocket leaves by washing and drying them thoroughly.

3. **Add Turkey and Greens:** Place the sliced turkey evenly across the wrap.
   - **American Standard:** Add spinach leaves over the turkey.
   - **British Touch:** Use rocket instead of spinach to introduce a peppery flavor that contrasts nicely with the sweet cranberry.

4. **Add Cranberry Sauce:** Spoon cranberry sauce over the turkey and greens, distributing it evenly for a burst of flavor in every bite.

5. **Roll the Wrap:** Carefully roll the wrap tightly, starting from the bottom and tucking in the sides as you go to keep all ingredients contained.

6. **Serve:** Cut the wrap in half diagonally to make it easier to handle and display the colorful contents. Serve immediately for the best freshness and taste.

Nutritional Information per Serving
- **Calories:** 380 kcal
- **Protein:** 20 g (40% of RDV)
- **Carbohydrates:** 45 g (17% of RDV)
- **Sugars:** 15 g (no daily recommended value for added sugars)
- **Fat:** 15 g (23% of RDV)
- **Saturated Fat:** 5 g (25% of RDV)
- **Fiber:** 5 g (20% of RDV)
- **Sodium:** 720 mg (31% of RDV)

28. GRILLED VEGGIE SANDWICH

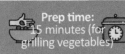 **Prep time:** 15 minutes (for grilling vegetables)   **Cooking time:** 5 minutes (for assembling and final heating if needed)   **Total time:** 20 minutes   **Servings:** 1

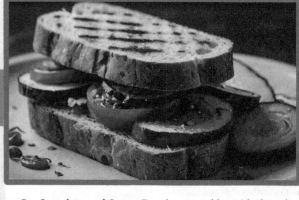

Ingredients

- **Grilled zucchini:** 1/4 cup, sliced
- **Bell peppers:** 1/4 cup, sliced
- **Eggplant:** 1/4 cup, sliced
- **Pesto:** 1 tbsp
- **Ciabatta bread:** 1 roll

American Twist:

- **Mozzarella cheese:** 2 slices

British Touch:

- **Beetroot hummus:** 2 tbsps

Step-by-Step Instructions

1. **Grill the Vegetables:** If not already grilled, lightly oil and grill slices of zucchini, bell peppers, and eggplant until they are tender and have grill marks, about 3-4 minutes per side.

2. **Prepare the Ciabatta:** Slice the ciabatta roll in half horizontally. Toast lightly if desired for added crunch.

3. **Spread Base:**
   - **American Standard:** Spread pesto on both halves of the ciabatta.
   - **British Touch:** Instead of pesto, spread beetroot hummus on both halves of the ciabatta for a sweet, earthy flavor contrast.

4. **Assemble the Sandwich:** Layer the grilled vegetables on the bottom half of the bread.
   - **American Twist:** Place mozzarella slices over the vegetables. If desired, place the sandwich under a broiler for a minute or two to melt the cheese and blend the flavors.
   - **British Version:** The beetroot hummus already adds a creamy texture, so additional cheese isn't necessary.

5. **Complete and Serve:** Top the vegetables with the other half of the ciabatta. Press down gently to compact the ingredients slightly. Cut the sandwich in half if desired and serve immediately.

Nutritional Information per Serving
- **Calories:** 450 kcal
- **Protein:** 15 g (30% of RDV)
- **Carbohydrates:** 55 g (21% of RDV)
- **Sugars:** 8 g (no daily recommended value for added sugars)
- **Fat:** 20 g (31% of RDV)
- **Saturated Fat:** 5 g (25% of RDV)
- **Fiber:** 6 g (24% of RDV)
- **Sodium:** 720 mg (31% of RDV)

29. CHICKEN CAESAR WRAP

 Prep time: 5 minutes **Cooking time:** Not Expected **Total time:** 5 minutes **Servings:** 1

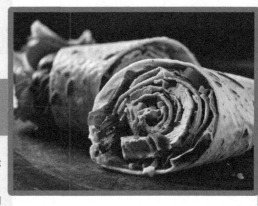

Ingredients
- **Sliced grilled chicken:** 1/2 cup
- **Romaine lettuce:** 1/2 cup, chopped
- **Whole wheat wrap:** 1
- **Caesar dressing:** 1 tbsp

American Twist:

- **Crumbled bacon:** 2 tbsps

British Touch:
- **Yogurt and mint dressing:** 1 tbsp (Mix 2 tsps plain yogurt with 1 tsp finely chopped mint, a squeeze of lemon juice, and a pinch of salt)

Step-by-Step Instructions

1. **Prepare the Wrap:** Lay the whole wheat wrap flat on a clean surface.

2. **Add Lettuce and Chicken:** Spread the chopped romaine lettuce evenly over the wrap, then layer the sliced grilled chicken on top.

3. **Standard:** Drizzle Caesar dressing over the chicken and lettuce for the classic flavor.

   - **American Twist:** After adding the Caesar dressing, sprinkle crumbled bacon over the chicken for a savory, crunchy addition that enhances the wrap with a typical American flair.
   - **British Touch:** Instead of Caesar dressing, spread the yogurt and mint dressing over the lettuce before adding the chicken. This lighter, refreshing dressing gives the wrap a distinctly British flavor, perfect for those seeking a healthier, herby alternative.

4. **Roll the Wrap:** Carefully roll the wrap tightly, starting from the bottom and tucking in the sides as you go to keep the ingredients contained.

5. **Serve:** Cut the wrap in half diagonally for easier handling and a display of the contents. Enjoy immediately for the best taste and texture.

Nutritional Information per Serving
- **Calories:** 350 kcal
- **Protein:** 25 g (50% of RDV)
- **Carbohydrates:** 30 g (11% of RDV)
- **Sugars:** 3 g (no daily recommended value for added sugars)
- **Fat:** 15 g (23% of RDV)
- **Saturated Fat:** 4 g (20% of RDV)
- **Fiber:** 4 g (16% of RDV)
- **Sodium:** 680 mg (29% of RDV)

30. TUNA STUFFED TOMATO

 Prep time: 10 minutes **Cooking time:** Not Expected **Total time:** 10 minutes **Servings:** 1

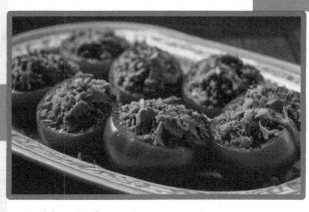

Ingredients
- **Canned tuna:** 1/2 cup, drained
- **Light mayonnaise:** 2 tbsps
- **Celery:** 1 tbsp, finely chopped
- **Onion:** 1 tbsp, finely chopped
- **Hollowed out tomatoes:** 2 medium

American Twist:

- **Chopped hard-boiled eggs:** 1, finely chopped

British Touch:

- **Capers:** 1 tsp
- **Cucumber:** 1 tbsp, finely diced

Step-by-Step Instructions

1. **Prepare the Tomatoes:** Carefully slice off the top of each tomato and use a spoon to hollow out the insides, removing the seeds and pulp to create a cavity for the filling. Set aside the hollowed-out tomatoes.

2. **Make Tuna Salad:** In a mixing bowl, combine the drained tuna, light mayonnaise, finely chopped celery, and onion. Mix until well combined.

   - **American Twist:** Add the chopped hard-boiled eggs to the tuna salad. The eggs provide additional protein and a rich texture that complements the tuna perfectly.
   - **British Touch:** Stir in capers and finely diced cucumber into the tuna mixture. Capers add a burst of tangy flavor, and the cucumber brings a refreshing crunch, enhancing the overall freshness of the dish.

3. **Stuff the Tomatoes:** Spoon the tuna salad mixture into each hollowed-out tomato, filling them generously.

4. **Serve:** Arrange the stuffed tomatoes on a plate. They can be served immediately or chilled in the refrigerator for about an hour before serving to enhance the flavors.

Nutritional Information per Serving
- **Calories:** 300 kcal
- **Protein:** 25 g (50% of RDV)
- **Carbohydrates:** 12 g (4% of RDV)
- **Sugars:** 6 g (no daily recommended value for added sugars)
- **Fat:** 18 g (28% of RDV)
- **Saturated Fat:** 3 g (15% of RDV)
- **Fiber:** 3 g (12% of RDV)
- **Sodium:** 480 mg (20% of RDV)

31. GREEK SALAD WITH CHICKEN

 Prep time: 10 minutes   **Cooking time:** Not Expected   **Total time:** 10 minutes   **Servings:** 1

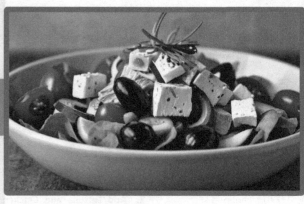

Ingredients

- **Chopped cucumber:** 1/2 cup
- **Tomatoes:** 1/2 cup, chopped
- **Red onion:** 1/4 cup, thinly sliced
- **Olives:** 1/4 cup, pitted and halved
- **Grilled chicken strips:** 1/2 cup
- **Feta cheese:** 1/4 cup, crumbled

American Twist:

- **Ranch dressing:** 2 tbsps, to drizzle

British Touch:

- **Pita bread:** 1 whole, to serve on the side

Step-by-Step Instructions

1. **Prepare the Salad:** In a large mixing bowl, combine the chopped cucumber, tomatoes, thinly sliced red onion, olives, and grilled chicken strips.

2. **Add Cheese:** Sprinkle the crumbled feta cheese over the salad mixture, adding a creamy texture and a salty flavor that complements the fresh vegetables and chicken.

3. **Dress the Salad:**

   • **American Twist:** Drizzle ranch dressing over the salad just before serving. The creamy and tangy flavors of the ranch dressing add a comforting American flair to the classic Greek salad.

4. **Serve:**

   • **British Touch:** Accompany the salad with a side of warm pita bread. The pita serves as a hearty addition, perfect for scooping up the salad and enjoying every bite.

5. **Enjoy:** Toss the salad lightly to mix all the ingredients and dressing, then serve immediately to ensure freshness and vibrant flavors.

Nutritional Information per Serving
- **Calories:** 400 kcal
- **Protein:** 30 g (60% of RDV)
- **Carbohydrates:** 30 g (11% of RDV)
- **Sugars:** 8 g (no daily recommended value for added sugars)
- **Fat:** 20 g (31% of RDV)
- **Saturated Fat:** 6 g (30% of RDV)
- **Fiber:** 4 g (16% of RDV)
- **Sodium:** 700 mg (30% of RDV)

32. SHRIMP AND AVOCADO SALAD

 Prep time: 10 minutes   **Cooking time:** Not Expected   **Total time:** 10 minutes   **Servings:** 1

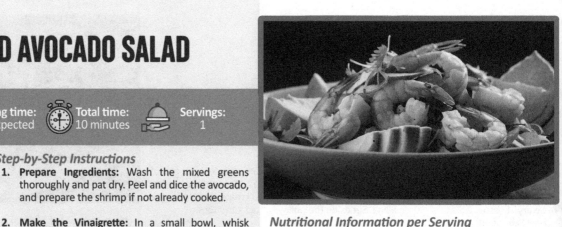

Ingredients
- **Cooked shrimp:** 1/2 cup
- **Diced avocado:** 1/2 of a medium avocado
- **Mixed greens:** 1 cup
- **Lime vinaigrette:** 2 tbsps (mix 1 tbsp olive oil, 1 tbsp lime juice, salt, and pepper)

American Twist:

- **Chili flakes:** A sprinkle, for garnish

British Touch:

- **Slices of mango:** 1/4 cup

Step-by-Step Instructions

1. **Prepare Ingredients:** Wash the mixed greens thoroughly and pat dry. Peel and dice the avocado, and prepare the shrimp if not already cooked.

2. **Make the Vinaigrette:** In a small bowl, whisk together olive oil, lime juice, salt, and pepper to create a refreshing lime vinaigrette.

3. **Assemble the Salad:** In a serving bowl, combine the mixed greens, cooked shrimp, and diced avocado.

   • **British Touch:** Add the slices of mango to the salad for a sweet, tropical flavor that complements the creamy texture of the avocado and the freshness of the shrimp.

4. **Dress the Salad:** Drizzle the lime vinaigrette over the salad and toss gently to coat all ingredients evenly.

   • **American Twist:** Sprinkle chili flakes over the salad for a mild heat and vibrant color that enhance the overall flavor profile.

5. **Serve:** Enjoy the salad immediately to ensure the avocado remains fresh and the greens crisp.

Nutritional Information per Serving
- **Calories:** 350 kcal
- **Protein:** 18 g (36% of RDV)
- **Carbohydrates:** 20 g (8% of RDV)
- **Sugars:** 5 g (no daily recommended value for added sugars)
- **Fat:** 25 g (38% of RDV)
- **Saturated Fat:** 3.5 g (17.5% of RDV)
- **Fiber:** 7 g (28% of RDV)
- **Sodium:** 300 mg (13% of RDV)

33. TOFU STIR-FRY

Prep time: 10 minutes **Cooking time:** 10 minutes **Total time:** 20 minutes **Servings:** 1

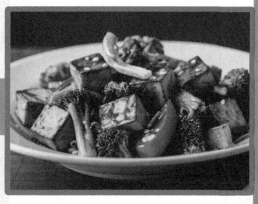

Ingredients
- **Firm tofu:** 1/2 cup, pressed and cubed
- **Mixed bell peppers:** 1/2 cup, sliced
- **Soy sauce:** 1 tbsp
- **Garlic:** 1 clove, minced
- **Sesame oil:** 1 tsp

American Twist:

- **Serve over brown rice:** 1/2 cup, cooked

British Touch:

- **Serve over cauliflower rice:** 1/2 cup, grated and sautéed

Step-by-Step Instructions
1. **Prepare Tofu:** Press the tofu to remove excess water for about 20 minutes before cooking. Then, cube the tofu to ensure even cooking.

2. **Cook Tofu and Vegetables:** Heat sesame oil in a large skillet or wok over medium-high heat. Add minced garlic and sauté until fragrant, about 1 minute. Add the cubed tofu and stir-fry until golden, about 5 minutes. Add the sliced bell peppers and continue to stir-fry until the vegetables are tender-crisp about 3-4 minutes.

3. **Season:** Drizzle soy sauce over the tofu and vegetables, stirring to coat evenly. Cook for an additional minute to allow the flavors to meld.

4. **Prepare Base:**
   - **American Twist:** If serving over brown rice, ensure the rice is cooked according to package instructions. Serve the stir-fried tofu and vegetables over a bed of warm brown rice.
   - **British Touch:** For the cauliflower rice, grate a portion of cauliflower and sauté in a pan with a little oil until it is lightly browned and tender, about 5-6 minutes. Serve the stir-fry over the prepared cauliflower rice for a low-carb alternative.

5. **Serve:** Plate the tofu stir-fry over your chosen base, garnishing with a sprinkle of sesame seeds or chopped green onions for added flavor and presentation.

Nutritional Information per Serving
- **Calories:** 350 kcal
- **Protein:** 18 g (36% of RDV)
- **Carbohydrates:** 45 g (17% of RDV)
- **Sugars:** 6 g (no daily recommended value for added sugars)
- **Fat:** 12 g (18% of RDV)
- **Saturated Fat:** 2 g (10% of RDV)
- **Fiber:** 6 g (24% of RDV)
- **Sodium:** 900 mg (39% of RDV)

34. CHICKPEA SALAD SANDWICH

Prep time: 10 minutes **Cooking time:** Not Expected **Total time:** 10 minutes **Servings:** 1

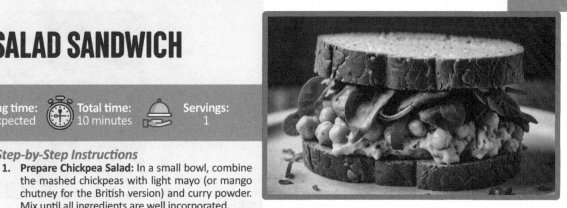

Ingredients
- **Mashed chickpeas:** 1/2 cup
- **Light mayonnaise:** 1 tbsp (substitute with mango chutney for the British touch)
- **Curry powder:** 1/2 tsp
- **Whole grain bread:** 2 slices

American Twist:

- **Raisins:** 1 tbsp, mixed into the chickpea salad

British Touch:

- **Mango chutney:** 1 tbsp, used instead of mayo

Step-by-Step Instructions
1. **Prepare Chickpea Salad:** In a small bowl, combine the mashed chickpeas with light mayo (or mango chutney for the British version) and curry powder. Mix until all ingredients are well incorporated.
   - **American Twist:** Stir in raisins with the chickpea mixture for a sweet contrast to the savory flavors.

2. **Assemble the Sandwich:** Lay out the slices of whole grain bread on a clean surface. Spread the chickpea salad evenly over one slice of bread.
   - **British Touch:** If using mango chutney, spread it on the inside of the second slice of bread for additional flavor and moisture.

3. **Complete the Sandwich:** Place the second slice of bread on top of the chickpea salad to form the sandwich.

4. **Serve:** Cut the sandwich in half diagonally and serve immediately. Optionally, you can toast the bread before assembling for added texture and warmth.

Nutritional Information per Serving
- **Calories:** 350 kcal
- **Protein:** 12 g (24% of RDV)
- **Carbohydrates:** 45 g (17% of RDV)
- **Sugars:** 10 g (no daily recommended value for added sugars)
- **Fat:** 12 g (18% of RDV)
- **Saturated Fat:** 1.5 g (7.5% of RDV)
- **Fiber:** 6 g (24% of RDV)
- **Sodium:** 500 mg (22% of RDV)

35. SEITAN AND PEPPER SKEWERS

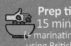 **Prep time:** 15 minutes (+ marinating time if using British touch)

 Cooking time: 10 minutes

Total time: 25 minutes

Servings: 1

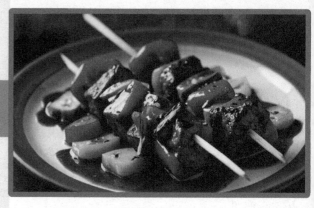

Ingredients

- **Seitan chunks:** 1 cup
- **Red peppers:** 1/2 cup, cut into 1-inch pieces
- **Yellow peppers:** 1/2 cup, cut into 1-inch pieces
- **Onions:** 1/2 cup, cut into 1-inch pieces
- **Barbecue sauce:** 2 tbsps

American Twist:
- **Honey-garlic sauce:** 2 tbsps, used for glazing

British Touch:
- **Apple cider vinegar and mustard marinade:** Mix 1 tbsp apple cider vinegar with 1 tsp mustard and 1 tsp olive oil

Step-by-Step Instructions

1. **Prepare the Marinade (for British Touch):** In a bowl, combine apple cider vinegar, mustard, and olive oil. Marinate the seitan chunks in this mixture for at least 30 minutes to infuse them with flavor.

2. **Assemble the Skewers:** Thread the marinated seitan chunks **(or plain if using American twist)**, red peppers, yellow peppers, and onions onto skewers. If using wooden skewers, soak them in water for at least 30 minutes beforehand to prevent burning.

3. **Prepare the Grill:** Preheat a grill or grill pan over medium heat. Ensure it's hot to get a good sear on the skewers.

4. **Grill the Skewers:** Grill the skewers, turning occasionally, until the vegetables are charred and the seitan is heated through, about 8-10 minutes. Brush with barbecue sauce during the last few minutes of grilling.

   • **Add American Twist:** If using the American twist, glaze the skewers with honey-garlic sauce during the last few minutes of cooking for a sweet and savory finish.

5. **Serve:** Serve the skewers hot off the grill. If using the British touch, any leftover marinade can be brushed over the skewers right before serving for extra flavor.

Nutritional Information per Serving
- **Calories:** 350 kcal
- **Protein:** 25 g (50% of RDV)
- **Carbohydrates:** 35 g (14% of RDV)
- **Sugars:** 15 g (no daily recommended value for added sugars)
- **Fat:** 10 g (15% of RDV)
- **Saturated Fat:** 1.5 g (7.5% of RDV)
- **Fiber:** 5 g (20% of RDV)
- **Sodium:** 700 mg (30% of RDV)

36. VEGAN CHILI

 Prep time: 10 minutes

 Cooking time: 25 minutes

 Total time: 35 minutes

 Servings: 1

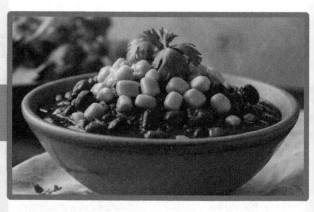

Ingredients

- **Black beans:** 1/2 cup, drained and rinsed
- **Kidney beans:** 1/2 cup, drained and rinsed
- **Tomatoes:** 1 cup, diced
- **Corn:** 1/2 cup
- **Chili spices (such as cumin, chili powder, and garlic powder):** 1 tsp

American Twist:
- **Avocado slices:** 1/4 avocado, sliced

British Touch:
- **Vegan sour cream:** 2 tbsps
- **Chives:** 1 tbsp, chopped

Step-by-Step Instructions

1. **Cook the Chili:** In a medium saucepan, combine the black beans, kidney beans, tomatoes, corn, and chili spices. Add a cup of water (adjust based on desired thickness) and stir well. Bring the mixture to a boil, then reduce the heat and simmer for about 20 minutes, or until the chili thickens and the flavors meld together.

   • **American Twist:** Just before serving, top the chili with avocado slices. The creamy texture of the avocado will contrast beautifully with the hearty and spicy chili, adding a refreshing touch that's popular in American cuisine.

   • **British Touch:** Serve the chili with a dollop of vegan sour cream on top. Sprinkle chopped chives over the sour cream for a burst of mild onion flavor. This addition not only adds a creamy texture but also visually enhances the dish, a common practice in British servings.

2. **Serve:** Ladle the hot chili into a bowl and apply the chosen topping based on the twist you're incorporating. Serve hot, ideally with a side of crusty bread or over a bed of rice for a more filling meal.

Nutritional Information per Serving
- **Calories:** 400 kcal
- **Protein:** 20 g (40% of RDV)
- **Carbohydrates:** 60 g (23% of RDV)
- **Sugars:** 10 g (no daily recommended value for added sugars)
- **Fat:** 10 g (15% of RDV)
- **Saturated Fat:** 1 g (5% of RDV)
- **Fiber:** 15 g (60% of RDV)
- **Sodium:** 500 mg (22% of RDV)

LUNCH – VEGAN/VEGETARIAN MEALS

37. GRILLED CHICKEN WITH ASPARAGUS

 Prep time: 10 minutes **Cooking time:** 15 minutes **Total time:** 25 minutes **Servings:** 1

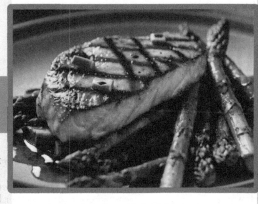

Ingredients
- **Chicken breast:** 1 (about 6 oz or 170 g)
- **Asparagus:** 1 cup, trimmed
- **Lemon zest:** 1 tsp

American Twist:
- **Smoked paprika:** 1/2 tsp

British Touch:
- **Mint yogurt sauce:** 2 tbsps (mix 2 tbsps plain yogurt with 1 tsp chopped fresh mint, a squeeze of lemon juice, and a pinch of salt)

Step-by-Step Instructions
1. **Prepare the Chicken and Asparagus:** Lightly coat the chicken breast and asparagus with olive oil. Sprinkle the chicken with lemon zest and season both the chicken and asparagus with salt and pepper to taste.

   - **American Twist:** Rub the smoked paprika all over the chicken breast before grilling. This will add a rich, smoky flavor that enhances the natural taste of the chicken.

2. **Grill the Chicken and Asparagus:** Preheat your grill to medium-high heat. Grill the chicken breast for about 6-7 minutes on each side or until fully cooked (internal temperature should reach 165°F or 74°C). Grill the asparagus alongside the chicken, turning occasionally, until tender and charred, about 5-7 minutes.

   - **Prepare the British Touch:** While the chicken and asparagus are grilling, prepare the mint yogurt sauce by mixing plain yogurt, chopped fresh mint, lemon juice, and a pinch of salt in a small bowl.

3. **Serve:** Plate the grilled chicken and asparagus.

   - **American Twist:** Serve as is, allowing the smoked paprika's robust flavor to stand out.
   - **British Touch:** Drizzle the mint yogurt sauce over the grilled chicken and asparagus for a refreshing, creamy contrast to the grilled flavors.

Nutritional Information per Serving
- **Calories:** 300 kcal
- **Protein:** 35 g (70% of RDV)
- **Carbohydrates:** 8 g (3% of RDV)
- **Sugars:** 3 g (no daily recommended value for added sugars)
- **Fat:** 15 g (23% of RDV)
- **Saturated Fat:** 2.5 g (12.5% of RDV)
- **Fiber:** 2 g (8% of RDV)
- **Sodium:** 200 mg (9% of RDV)

38. GRILLED SALMON WITH FENNEL SALAD

 Prep time: 10 minutes  **Cooking time:** 10 minutes **Total time:** 20 minutes **Servings:** 1

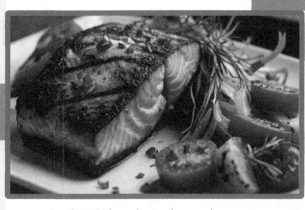

Ingredients
- **Salmon fillet:** 1 (about 6 oz or 170g)
- **Sliced fennel:** 1/2 cup
- **Arugula:** 1 cup
- **Lemon dressing:** 2 tbsps (mix 2 tsps olive oil, 1 tbsp lemon juice, salt, and pepper to taste)

American Twist:
- **Balsamic glaze:** 1 tbsp, for drizzling

British Touch:
- **Orange segments:** 1/4 cup, freshly segmented

Step-by-Step Instructions
1. **Prepare the Salad:** In a salad bowl, combine the sliced fennel and arugula. Toss with lemon dressing to coat evenly.

2. **Grill the Salmon:** Preheat your grill to medium-high heat. Lightly oil the grill grate. Season the salmon fillet with salt and pepper, then place it skin-side down on the grill. Cook for about 4-5 minutes per side or until the salmon is opaque and flakes easily with a fork.

   - **American Twist:** Just before serving, drizzle the salmon with balsamic glaze. The glaze will add a sweet and tangy flavor that complements the fatty richness of the salmon.
   - **British Touch:** If opting for the British touch, add orange segments to the fennel and arugula salad. The citrus adds a refreshing sweetness and vibrant color, enhancing the dish's overall appeal.

3. **Serve:** Arrange the salad on a plate. Place the grilled salmon on top of the salad.

   - For the **American version**, ensure the balsamic glaze is visibly drizzled over the salmon.
   - For the **British version**, make sure the orange segments are well distributed throughout the salad for bursts of flavor.

Nutritional Information per Serving
- **Calories:** 400 kcal
- **Protein:** 35 g (70% of RDV)
- **Carbohydrates:** 12 g (4% of RDV)
- **Sugars:** 7 g (no daily recommended value for added sugars)
- **Fat:** 25 g (38% of RDV)
- **Saturated Fat:** 4.5 g (22.5% of RDV)
- **Fiber:** 3 g (12% of RDV)
- **Sodium:** 300 mg (13% of RDV)

39. BEEF SKEWERS WITH BELL PEPPERS

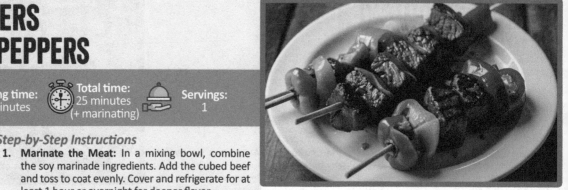

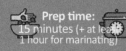 **Prep time:** 15 minutes (+ at least 1 hour for marinating) **Cooking time:** 10 minutes **Total time:** 25 minutes (+ marinating) **Servings:** 1

Ingredients

- **Lean beef:** 1 cup, cubed (about 170 g)
- **Bell peppers:** 1 cup, cut into 1-inch pieces
- **Onions:** 1/2 cup, cut into 1-inch pieces
- **Soy marinade:** 3 tbsps (combine soy sauce, a splash of olive oil, minced garlic, and a tsp of honey)

American Twist:
- **BBQ sauce:** 2 tbsps, for serving

British Touch:
- **Horseradish cream:** 2 tbsps, for serving

Step-by-Step Instructions

1. **Marinate the Meat:** In a mixing bowl, combine the soy marinade ingredients. Add the cubed beef and toss to coat evenly. Cover and refrigerate for at least 1 hour or overnight for deeper flavor.

2. **Assemble the Skewers:** If using wooden skewers, soak them in water for at least 30 minutes prior to grilling to prevent burning. Thread the marinated beef, bell peppers, and onions alternately onto the skewers.

3. **Grill the Skewers:** Preheat the grill to medium-high heat. Place the skewers on the grill, turning occasionally, until the beef is cooked to your liking and the vegetables are tender and slightly charred, about 8-10 minutes.

4. **Prepare Serving Sauces:**

   - **American Twist:** Have BBQ sauce ready for dipping or brushing over the cooked skewers.
   - **British Touch:** Prepare horseradish cream by mixing prepared horseradish with cream or sour cream, seasoned with a pinch of salt.

5. **Serve:** Plate the skewers hot off the grill.

   - **American Twist:** Serve with a side of BBQ sauce for a classic American BBQ experience.
   - **British Touch:** Serve with a dollop of horseradish cream on the side for a sharp, tangy complement that cuts through the richness of the beef.

Nutritional Information per Serving
- **Calories:** 400 kcal
- **Protein:** 35 g (70% of RDV)
- **Carbohydrates:** 15 g (6% of RDV)
- **Sugars:** 10 g (no daily recommended value for added sugars)
- **Fat:** 20 g (31% of RDV)
- **Saturated Fat:** 5 g (25% of RDV)
- **Fiber:** 2 g (8% of RDV)
- **Sodium:** 800 mg (35% of RDV)

40. GRILLED TOFU STEAKS WITH ZUCCHINI RIBBONS

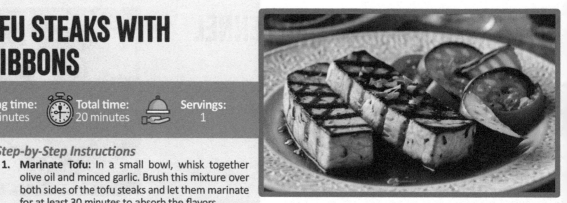

 Prep time: 10 minutes **Cooking time:** 10 minutes **Total time:** 20 minutes **Servings:** 1

Ingredients

- **Tofu:** 1 block (about 8 oz or 225 g), pressed and sliced into steaks
- **Zucchini:** 2 medium, sliced into thin ribbons using a vegetable peeler or mandoline
- **Olive oil:** 2 tbsps
- **Garlic:** 1 clove, minced

American Twist:
- **Chili flakes:** A sprinkle, for garnish

British Touch:
- **Pea puree:** 1/2 cup (blend cooked peas with a splash of olive oil, lemon juice, and mint for freshness)

Step-by-Step Instructions

1. **Marinate Tofu:** In a small bowl, whisk together olive oil and minced garlic. Brush this mixture over both sides of the tofu steaks and let them marinate for at least 30 minutes to absorb the flavors.

2. **Prepare Zucchini Ribbons:** Using a vegetable peeler or mandoline, slice the zucchini into thin ribbons. Lightly toss the ribbons with a bit of olive oil and a pinch of salt.

3. **Grill Tofu and Zucchini:** Preheat the grill to medium-high heat. Grill the tofu steaks for about 3-4 minutes per side, or until grill marks appear and the tofu is heated through. Grill the zucchini ribbons briefly, just until tender and lightly charred, about 1-2 minutes per side.

   - **American Twist:** Sprinkle chili flakes over the grilled tofu steaks for a spicy kick that complements the subtle flavors of the dish.
   - **Prepare British Touch:** If making pea puree, blend cooked peas with olive oil, lemon juice, and a little mint until smooth. Season with salt and pepper to taste.

4. **Serve:** Arrange the grilled tofu steaks and zucchini ribbons on a plate.

   - **American Twist:** Serve with chili flakes sprinkled on top for a vibrant flavor contrast.
   - **British Touch:** Serve the tofu and zucchini with a side of pea puree for a creamy, refreshing accompaniment that enhances the light and healthy nature of the meal.

Nutritional Information per Serving
- **Calories:** 400 kcal
- **Protein:** 25 g (50% of RDV)
- **Carbohydrates:** 15 g (5% of RDV)
- **Sugars:** 6 g (no daily recommended value for added sugars)
- **Fat:** 25 g (38% of RDV)
- **Saturated Fat:** 3 g (15% of RDV)
- **Fiber:** 6 g (24% of RDV)
- **Sodium:** 100 mg (4% of RDV)

41. CHICKEN AVOCADO SALAD

 Prep time: 10 minutes   **Cooking time:** Not Expected   **Total time:** 10 minutes   **Servings:** 1

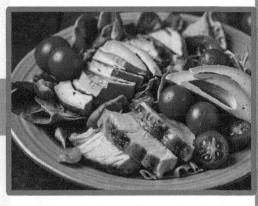

Ingredients
- **Grilled chicken:** 1/2 cup, sliced
- **Avocado:** 1/2, sliced
- **Mixed greens:** 1 cup
- **Cherry tomatoes:** 1/4 cup, halved
- **Vinaigrette:** 2 tbsps (combine olive oil, balsamic vinegar, a touch of honey, salt, and pepper)

American Twist:

- **Ranch dressing:** 2 tbsps to toss the salad

British Touch:
- **Watercress:** 1/4 cup, included with mixed greens

Step-by-Step Instructions
1. **Prepare the Salad Components:** Wash and dry the mixed greens and watercress. Slice the grilled chicken and avocado. Halve the cherry tomatoes.

2. **Assemble the Salad:** In a large mixing bowl, combine the mixed greens (and watercress for the British version), sliced avocado, cherry tomatoes, and grilled chicken.

3. **Dress the Salad:**
   - **Standard Version:** Drizzle the vinaigrette over the salad and toss gently to coat all the ingredients evenly.
   - **American Twist:** Instead of vinaigrette, use ranch dressing to toss the salad. The creamy texture and tangy flavor of the ranch dressing add a comforting American flair to the dish.

4. **Serve:** Plate the salad immediately after dressing to ensure the leaves remain crisp and the flavors are fresh.
   - **British Touch:** Ensure the watercress is well integrated throughout the salad for a peppery bite that complements the creamy avocado and savory chicken.

Nutritional Information per Serving
- **Calories:** 400 kcal
- **Protein:** 25 g (50% of RDV)
- **Carbohydrates:** 18 g (7% of RDV)
- **Sugars:** 4 g (no daily recommended value for added sugars)
- **Fat:** 28 g (43% of RDV)
- **Saturated Fat:** 4.5 g (22.5% of RDV)
- **Fiber:** 7 g (28% of RDV)
- **Sodium:** 300 mg (13% of RDV)

42. SHRIMP AND MANGO SALAD

 Prep time: 10 minutes   **Cooking time:** Not Expected   **Total time:** 10 minutes   **Servings:** 1

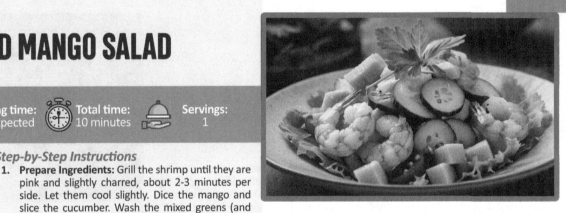

Ingredients
- **Grilled shrimp:** 1/2 cup
- **Mango:** 1/2, diced
- **Cucumber:** 1/4 cup, sliced
- **Mixed greens:** 1 cup
- **Lime dressing:** 2 tbsps (mix 2 tsps olive oil, 1 tbsp lime juice, a pinch of salt, and pepper)

American Twist:

- **Cilantro:** 1 tbsp, chopped

British Touch:
- **Rocket leaves:** 1/4 cup, mixed with the greens

Step-by-Step Instructions
1. **Prepare Ingredients:** Grill the shrimp until they are pink and slightly charred, about 2-3 minutes per side. Let them cool slightly. Dice the mango and slice the cucumber. Wash the mixed greens (and rocket leaves if using the British touch).

2. **Assemble the Salad:** In a large salad bowl, combine the mixed greens (including rocket leaves for the British version), diced mango, sliced cucumber, and grilled shrimp.

3. **Add Regional Twists:**
   - **American Twist:** Sprinkle chopped cilantro over the salad for a fresh, herby flavor that complements the sweetness of the mango and the tanginess of the lime dressing.
   - **British Touch:** The inclusion of rocket leaves adds a peppery flavor that contrasts delightfully with the sweet mango and crisp cucumber.

4. **Dress the Salad:** Drizzle the lime dressing over the salad and toss gently to ensure all ingredients are well coated.

5. **Serve:** Plate the salad and serve immediately to maintain the freshness of the ingredients and the crispness of the greens.

Nutritional Information per Serving
- **Calories:** 350 kcal
- **Protein:** 20 g (40% of RDV)
- **Carbohydrates:** 25 g (10% of RDV)
- **Sugars:** 15 g (no daily recommended value for added sugars)
- **Fat:** 15 g (23% of RDV)
- **Saturated Fat:** 2 g (10% of RDV)
- **Fiber:** 4 g (16% of RDV)
- **Sodium:** 200 mg (9% of RDV)

43. TUNA AND BEAN SALAD

 Prep time: 10 minutes   **Cooking time:** Not Expected   **Total time:** 10 minutes   **Servings:** 1

Ingredients
- **Canned tuna:** 1/2 cup, drained and flaked
- **Mixed beans (such as kidney, chickpea, and black beans):** 1 cup, rinsed and drained
- **Red onion:** 1/4 cup, finely chopped
- **Parsley:** 2 tbsps, chopped
- **Lemon vinaigrette:** 2 tbsps (mix 2 tsps olive oil, 1 tbsp lemon juice, salt, and pepper to taste)

American Twist:
- **Chopped dill pickles:** 2 tbsps

British Touch:
- **Capers:** 1 tbsp

Step-by-Step Instructions
1. **Prepare Ingredients:** In a large mixing bowl, combine the drained and flaked tuna, rinsed mixed beans, finely chopped red onion, and chopped parsley.

2. **Add Regional Twists:**

   • **American Twist:** Stir in chopped dill pickles into the salad mixture. The pickles add a tangy crunch that complements the creamy texture of the beans and the richness of the tuna.
   • **British Touch:** Mix in capers with the other ingredients. Capers provide a burst of salty, briny flavor that enhances the overall freshness of the salad.

3. **Dress the Salad:** Drizzle lemon vinaigrette over the salad and toss gently to coat all ingredients evenly. The lemon vinaigrette adds a bright, citrusy note that ties all the flavors together beautifully.

4. **Serve:** Plate the salad and serve immediately, or chill in the refrigerator for about an hour to let the flavors meld together even more, which can deepen the taste experience.

Nutritional Information per Serving
- **Calories:** 350 kcal
- **Protein:** 25 g (50% of RDV)
- **Carbohydrates:** 30 g (11% of RDV)
- **Sugars:** 4 g (no daily recommended value for added sugars)
- **Fat:** 15 g (23% of RDV)
- **Saturated Fat:** 2 g (10% of RDV)
- **Fiber:** 8 g (32% of RDV)
- **Sodium:** 600 mg (26% of RDV)

44. TOFU AND KALE SALAD

 Prep time: 15 minutes   **Cooking time:** Not Expected   **Total time:** 15 minutes   **Servings:** 1

Ingredients
- **Baked tofu:** 1/2 cup, cubed
- **Kale:** 1 cup, chopped and massaged
- **Avocado:** 1/2, diced
- **Sunflower seeds:** 2 tbsps
- **Sesame dressing:** 2 tbsps (mix 2 tsps sesame oil, 1 tbsp soy sauce, 1 tsp honey, and a splash of rice vinegar)

American Twist:
- **Sriracha:** 1 tbsp, for drizzling

British Touch:
- **Beetroot slices:** 1/4 cup, pre-cooked and sliced

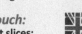

Step-by-Step Instructions
1. **Prepare the Salad Components:** Ensure the kale is washed, dried, and roughly chopped. Massage the kale with a little olive oil and a pinch of salt to soften its texture and enhance its flavor. Cube the baked tofu and dice the avocado.

2. **Assemble the Salad:** In a large salad bowl, combine the massaged kale, cubed baked tofu, diced avocado, and sunflower seeds.

   • **British Touch:** If using beetroot slices, add them to the salad now. The beetroot not only adds vibrant color but also introduces a sweet, earthy flavor that complements the creamy avocado and nutty sunflower seeds.

3. **Dress the Salad:** Drizzle sesame dressing over the salad and toss gently to ensure all ingredients are evenly coated.

4. **Add Regional Twists:**

   • **American Twist:** Just before serving, drizzle Sriracha over the salad for a bold, spicy kick that contrasts with the sesame dressing's subtle sweetness.

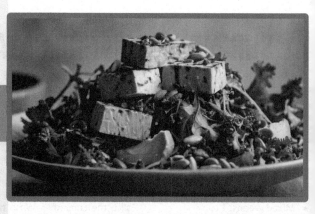

5. **Serve:** Plate the salad, ensuring if using the British touch, the beetroot slices are visibly distributed throughout. If opting for the American twist, make sure the Sriracha drizzle is evident for a visually appealing presentation.

Nutritional Information per Serving
- **Calories:** 400 kcal
- **Protein:** 15 g (30% of RDV)
- **Carbohydrates:** 25 g (10% of RDV)
- **Sugars:** 6 g (no daily recommended value for added sugars)
- **Fat:** 28 g (43% of RDV)
- **Saturated Fat:** 3 g (15% of RDV)
- **Fiber:** 7 g (28% of RDV)
- **Sodium:** 300 mg (13% of RDV)

45. GRILLED LEMON-HERB CHICKEN SALAD

 Prep time: 10 minutes   **Cooking time:** 10 minutes   **Total time:** 20 minutes   **Servings:** 1

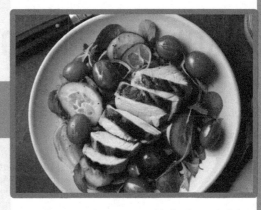

Ingredients

- **Chicken breast, boneless & skinless:** 1 small (about 120g)
- **Mixed salad greens:** 1 cup (30 g)
- **Cherry tomatoes, halved:** 1/4 cup (50 g)
- **Cucumber, sliced:** 1/4 cup (30 g)
- **Lemon juice:** 1 tbsp
- **Olive oil:** 1 tsp
- **Fresh herbs (parsley, thyme, basil), chopped:** 1 tbsp
- **Salt and pepper:** to taste

American Touch:
- **Dried cranberries:** 1 tbsp

British Touch:
- **Stilton cheese, crumbled:** 1 tbsp

Step-by-Step Instructions

1. **Marinate the Chicken:** In a small bowl, combine half of the lemon juice, half of the olive oil, half of the chopped herbs, and salt and pepper. Add the chicken breast and let marinate for at least 15 minutes.

2. **Grill the Chicken:** Preheat a grill or skillet over medium heat. Grill the chicken for about 5 minutes on each side or until fully cooked and internal temperature reaches 165°F (74°C). Remove from heat and let it rest for a few minutes before slicing.

3. **Prepare the Salad:** In a large bowl, combine the mixed salad greens, cherry tomatoes, and cucumber slices.
   - **American Touch:** Add dried cranberries to the salad for a sweet, tangy flavor.
   - **British Touch:** Crumble Stilton cheese over the salad for a rich and creamy texture.

4. **Dressing:** In a small bowl, whisk together the remaining lemon juice, olive oil, herbs, and season with salt and pepper to taste. Drizzle over the salad.

5. **Assemble:** Add the sliced chicken to the salad and toss gently to combine.

6. **Serve:** Enjoy your meal fresh and light, perfect for a nutritious lunch or dinner.

Tips and Variations
- **More Protein:** Add a hard-boiled egg or a scoop of quinoa to the salad for extra protein.
- **Low-Fat Option:** Substitute olive oil with a splash of apple cider vinegar for a lower-fat dressing option.

Storage and Serving Suggestions
- **Freshness:** This salad is best enjoyed fresh, however, if needed, you can refrigerate the grilled chicken for up to 2 days. Assemble the salad just before serving to maintain crispness.

Nutritional Information per Serving
- **Calories:** 250 kcal -**Protein:** 28 g (56% of RDV)
- **Carbohydrates:** 12 g (4%) -**Sugars:** 6 g
- **Fat:** 10 g (15%) -**Saturated Fat:** 2.5 g (12.5%)
- **Fiber:** 2 g (8%) - **Sodium:** 200mg (8.3%)

46. CUCUMBER AND TURKEY ROLL-UPS

 Prep time: 10 minutes   **Cooking time:** Not Expected   **Total time:** 10 minutes   **Servings:** 1

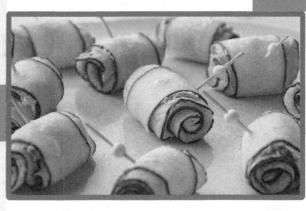

Ingredients

- **Cucumber, large, thinly sliced lengthwise:** 1 (about 200 g)
- **Deli turkey breast, thinly sliced:** 4 slices (about 100 g)

American Touch: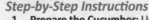
- **Light cream cheese:** 2 tbsps (30 g)

British Touch:
- **Mustard, preferably Dijon or English:** 1 tbsp (15 ml)

Step-by-Step Instructions

1. **Prepare the Cucumber:** Using a mandoline slicer or a sharp knife, carefully slice the cucumber lengthwise into thin strips. Aim for slices that are flexible but sturdy enough to hold the filling without breaking.

2. **Add the Flavors:**
   - **American Twist:** Spread a thin layer of light cream cheese over each turkey slice. This adds creaminess and helps the cucumber stick to the turkey.
   - **British Touch:** Lightly brush mustard on top of the cream cheese for a tangy kick.

3. **Assemble the Roll-ups:** Lay a strip of cucumber on a flat surface. Place a slice of turkey with cream cheese and mustard on top of the cucumber, aligning it at one end of the cucumber strip.

4. **Roll Up:** Carefully roll the cucumber around the turkey, starting from the end where the turkey is placed. Roll tightly to ensure the filling stays in place.

5. **Serve:** Arrange the roll-ups on a plate. They can be served whole or sliced into smaller pieces to make bite-sized appetizers.

Tips and Variations
- **Additional Fillings:** Include a slice of avocado or a sprinkle of chopped herbs like dill or chives inside the roll-ups for added flavor and texture.
- **Vegan Option:** Substitute turkey with a plant-based deli slice and use vegan cream cheese.

Storage and Serving Suggestions
- **Immediate Consumption:** These roll-ups are best enjoyed soon after making to ensure the cucumber remains crisp.
- **Prep Ahead:** You can prepare the turkey with cream cheese and mustard in advance, but slice and assemble the cucumber just before serving to maintain freshness.

Nutritional Information per Serving
- **Calories:** 150 kcal - **Protein:** 18 g (36% of RDV)
- **Carbohydrates:** 6 g (2%)
- **Sugars:** 3 g | Fat: 6 g (9%) - **Saturated Fat:** 2 g (10%)
- **Fiber:** 1 g (4%) - **Sodium:** 850 mg (35.4%)

47. CHICKEN MINESTRONE SOUP

 Prep time: 10 minutes **Cooking time:** 30 minutes **Total time:** 40 minutes **Servings:** 1

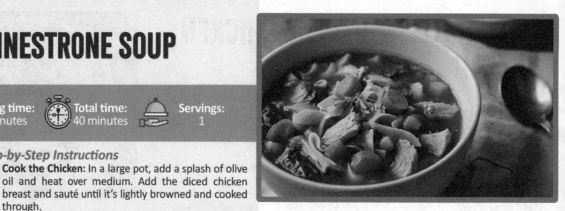

Ingredients
- **Chicken breast:** 1/2 cup, diced
- **Carrots:** 1/4 cup, diced
- **Celery:** 1/4 cup, diced
- **Tomatoes:** 1/2 cup, diced
- **Zucchini:** 1/4 cup, diced
- **Chicken broth:** 2 cups

American Twist:
- **Macaroni pasta:** 1/4 cup, uncooked

British Touch: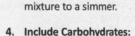
- **Pearl barley:** 1/4 cup, rinsed

Step-by-Step Instructions
1. **Cook the Chicken:** In a large pot, add a splash of olive oil and heat over medium. Add the diced chicken breast and sauté until it's lightly browned and cooked through.

2. **Add Vegetables:** To the pot with the chicken, add the diced carrots, celery, tomatoes, and zucchini. Cook for about 5 minutes, stirring occasionally, until the vegetables begin to soften.

3. **Add Liquid:** Pour in the chicken broth and bring the mixture to a simmer.

4. **Include Carbohydrates:**

   • **American Twist:** Add the macaroni pasta to the simmering soup. Cook according to the package instructions, typically about 8-10 minutes, until tender.
   • **British Touch:** Add the rinsed pearl barley at the same time as the chicken broth. Allow the soup to simmer for about 25 minutes, or until the barley is fully cooked and tender.

5. **Season and Serve:** Season the soup with salt and pepper to taste. Let it simmer for a final 5 minutes to meld all the flavors together.

• Serve the soup hot, ensuring that if using the **American twist**, the pasta is cooked just right, or if using the **British touch**, the barley has softened and thickened the soup slightly.

Nutritional Information per Serving
- **Calories:** 350 kcal
- **Protein:** 30 g (60% of RDV)
- **Carbohydrates:** 35 g (14% of RDV)
- **Sugars:** 6 g (no daily recommended value for added sugars)
- **Fat:** 10 g (15% of RDV)
- **Saturated Fat:** 2 g (10% of RDV)
- **Fiber:** 6 g (24% of RDV)
- **Sodium:** 700 mg (30% of RDV)

48. BEEF AND VEGETABLE SOUP

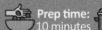 **Prep time:** 10 minutes **Cooking time:** 30 minutes **Total time:** 40 minutes **Servings:** 1

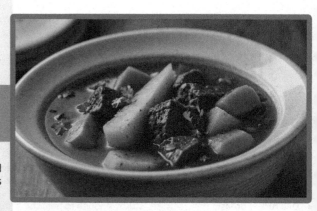

Ingredients
- **Lean beef:** 1/2 cup, cubed
- **Potatoes:** 1/2 cup, cubed
- **Carrots:** 1/4 cup, sliced
- **Beef broth:** 2 cups
- **Peas:** 1/4 cup

American Twist:
- **Light sour cream:** 1 tbsp, for serving

British Touch:
- **Worcestershire sauce:** 1 tsp, mixed into the broth

Step-by-Step Instructions
1. **Prepare the Ingredients:** Cube the lean beef and potatoes. Slice the carrots. Have all your vegetables prepped and ready.

2. **Cook the Beef:** In a large pot, heat a drizzle of oil over medium heat. Add the beef cubes and sauté until browned on all sides.

3. **Add Vegetables and Broth:** To the pot, add the potatoes, carrots, and beef broth. Bring to a simmer.

   • **British Touch:** Stir in Worcestershire sauce into the broth for a deep, savory flavor that enhances the overall taste of the soup.
4. **Simmer:** Let the soup simmer for about 20 minutes, or until the beef and vegetables are tender. About 5 minutes before the end of cooking, add the peas to cook through.

5. **Season and Serve:** Adjust the seasoning with salt and pepper to taste.

   • **American Twist:** Serve the soup hot with a dollop of light sour cream on top. The sour cream adds a creamy texture and a slight tang, providing a rich contrast to the hearty soup.

Nutritional Information per Serving
- **Calories:** 350 kcal
- **Protein:** 30 g (60% of RDV)
- **Carbohydrates:** 30 g (11% of RDV)
- **Sugars:** 5 g (no daily recommended value for added sugars)
- **Fat:** 10 g (15% of RDV)
- **Saturated Fat:** 3 g (15% of RDV)
- **Fiber:** 4 g (16% of RDV)
- **Sodium:** 800 mg (35% of RDV)

49. LENTIL AND SPINACH SOUP

 Prep time: 10 minutes **Cooking time:** 30 minutes **Total time:** 40 minutes **Servings:** 1

Ingredients
- **Lentils:** 1/2 cup, rinsed and drained
- **Spinach:** 1 cup, roughly chopped
- **Carrots:** 1/4 cup, diced
- **Onions:** 1/4 cup, diced
- **Vegetable broth:** 2 cups

American Twist:
- **Smoked turkey sausage:** 1/2 cup, sliced

British Touch:
- **Curry powder:** 1 tsp

Step-by-Step Instructions
1. **Cook the Lentils:** Add the rinsed lentils and vegetable broth to a large pot. Bring to a boil, then reduce the heat to a simmer. Cook until the lentils are tender, about 20 minutes.

2. **Prepare Vegetables and Additions:** While the lentils are cooking, heat a small amount of oil in a pan over medium heat. Sauté the onions and carrots until they are soft, about 5 minutes.
   - **American Twist:** Add sliced smoked turkey sausage to the pan and sauté until browned, adding a rich, smoky flavor to the soup.
   - **British Touch:** Stir curry powder into the onion and carrot mixture, cooking briefly to release the aromatic flavors.

3. **Combine Ingredients:**
   - Add the sautéed vegetables (and sausage if using the American twist) to the simmering lentils.
   - Stir in the chopped spinach during the last 5 minutes of cooking, allowing it to wilt but retain its vibrant green color.

4. **Season and Serve:**
   - Adjust the seasoning with salt and pepper to taste.
   - Serve the soup hot, ensuring that the flavors have melded together beautifully. The distinct addition of either smoked turkey sausage or curry powder enhances the traditional lentil and spinach soup base.

Nutritional Information per Serving
- **Calories:** 350 kcal
- **Protein:** 25 g (50% of RDV)
- **Carbohydrates:** 40 g (15% of RDV)
- **Sugars:** 5 g (no daily recommended value for added sugars)
- **Fat:** 10 g (15% of RDV)
- **Saturated Fat:** 2 g (10% of RDV)
- **Fiber:** 15 g (60% of RDV)
- **Sodium:** 700 mg (30% of RDV)

50. SEAFOOD CHOWDER

 Prep time: 10 minutes **Cooking time:** 20 minutes **Total time:** 30 minutes **Servings:** 1

Ingredients
- **Mixed seafood (such as shrimp, scallops, and clams):** 1 cup
- **Potatoes:** 1/2 cup, diced
- **Onions:** 1/4 cup, finely chopped
- **Fish broth:** 2 cups
- **Light cream:** 1/2 cup

American Twist:
- **Corn kernels:** 1/4 cup

British Touch:
- **Saffron:** A pinch

Step-by-Step Instructions
1. **Prepare the Base:** In a large pot, sauté the onions in a bit of butter or oil until translucent. Add the diced potatoes and cook for a few minutes until slightly tender.

2. **Cook the Seafood:** Add the mixed seafood to the pot. Pour in the fish broth and bring to a simmer. Allow the seafood to cook just until it's done, which typically takes about 5-7 minutes depending on the size and type of seafood.

3. **Add Cream and Flavors:** Reduce the heat to low and stir in the light cream.
   - **American Twist:** Stir in the corn kernels for a sweet pop of flavor and texture, a common addition in American-style chowders.
   - **British Touch:** Add a pinch of saffron for a luxurious aroma and a rich golden color, enhancing the chowder with a sophisticated British flair.

4. **Simmer and Serve:** Allow the chowder to simmer gently for another 5-10 minutes to let all the flavors meld together. Be careful not to let it boil to prevent the cream from curdling. Season with salt and pepper to taste.

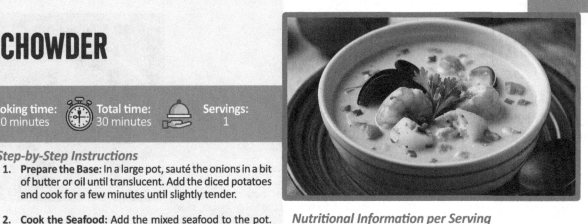

Nutritional Information per Serving
- **Calories:** 450 kcal
- **Protein:** 25 g (50% of RDV)
- **Carbohydrates:** 38 g (14% of RDV)
- **Sugars:** 5 g (no daily recommended value for added sugars)
- **Fat:** 20 g (31% of RDV)
- **Saturated Fat:** 10 g (50% of RDV)
- **Fiber:** 4 g (16% of RDV)
- **Sodium:** 950 mg (41% of RDV)

51. CHICKEN AND BROCCOLI BAKE

 Prep time: 15 minutes   **Cooking time:** 30 minutes  **Total time:** 45 minutes   **Servings:** 1

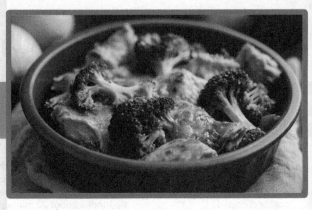

Ingredients

- **Chicken breast:** 1 cup, diced
- **Broccoli:** 1 cup, chopped
- **Low-fat cheese:** 1/2 cup, grated
- **Whole wheat breadcrumbs:** 1/4 cup

American Twist:

- **Sweet potato mash:** 1/2 cup, spread as a layer

British Touch:

- **Leeks:** 1/4 cup, finely sliced and mixed in

Step-by-Step Instructions

1. **Preheat Oven:** Preheat your oven to 375°F (190°C).

2. **Prepare Ingredients:**

   - Steam or boil the broccoli until it's just tender, about 3-4 minutes.
   - If including sweet potato mash **(American twist)**, peel, boil, and mash sweet potatoes with a little salt and pepper.
   - Cook the chicken pieces in a pan over medium heat until fully cooked.

3. **Combine Ingredients:**

   - In a baking dish, layer the cooked chicken and broccoli. If using the **British touch**, mix in finely sliced leeks with the chicken and broccoli.
   - **American Twist:** Spread a layer of sweet potato mash over the chicken and broccoli.
   - Sprinkle grated low-fat cheese over the top and then cover with whole wheat breadcrumbs for a crispy topping.

4. **Bake:** Place the baking dish in the oven and bake for 20-25 minutes, or until the top is golden brown and everything is heated through.

5. **Serve:** Remove from the oven and let cool slightly before serving. This dish is great on its own or can be served with a side salad for added freshness.

Nutritional Information per Serving

- **Calories:** 500 kcal
- **Protein:** 40 g (80% of RDV)
- **Carbohydrates:** 40 g (15% of RDV)
- **Sugars:** 5 g (no daily recommended value for added sugars)
- **Fat:** 20 g (31% of RDV)
- **Saturated Fat:** 5 g (25% of RDV)
- **Fiber:** 7 g (28% of RDV)
- **Sodium:** 400 mg (17% of RDV)

52. TURKEY SHEPHERD'S PIE

 Prep time: 15 minutes   **Cooking time:** 30 minutes   **Total time:** 45 minutes   **Servings:** 1

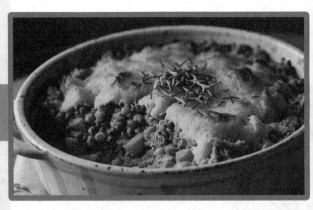

Ingredients

- **Ground turkey:** 1/2 cup
- **Carrots:** 1/4 cup, diced
- **Peas:** 1/4 cup
- **Mashed cauliflower topping:** 1 cup (steamed cauliflower mashed with a bit of olive oil, salt, and pepper)

American Twist:

- **Celery:** 1/4 cup, diced

British Touch:

- **Parsnip:** 1/4 cup, diced and mixed into the cauliflower mash

Step-by-Step Instructions

1. **Preheat Oven:** Preheat your oven to 375°F (190°C).

2. **Prepare the Base:** In a skillet over medium heat, cook the ground turkey until it's no longer pink. Add the diced carrots, peas, and celery (**if using the American twist**). Cook for about 5-7 minutes, until the vegetables are tender.

3. **Prepare the Topping:** For the cauliflower mash, steam the cauliflower until tender. Mash it with a bit of olive oil, salt, and pepper.

   - **British Touch:** Steam parsnip along with the cauliflower. Mash them together for a slightly sweet flavor that complements the turkey.

4. **Assemble the Pie:**

   - Spoon the turkey and vegetable mixture into a small baking dish.
   - Spread the mashed cauliflower (and parsnip, if using the British touch) over the top, smoothing it into an even layer.

5. **Bake:** Place the pie in the preheated oven and bake for 20-25 minutes, or until the topping is slightly golden and the edges are bubbly.

6. **Serve:** Let the pie cool for a few minutes before serving. This ensures that it sets slightly and makes it easier to serve.

Nutritional Information per Serving

- **Calories:** 400 kcal
- **Protein:** 35 g (70% of RDV)
- **Carbohydrates:** 25 g (10% of RDV)
- **Sugars:** 8 g (no daily recommended value for added sugars)
- **Fat:** 15 g (23% of RDV)
- **Saturated Fat:** 3 g (15% of RDV)
- **Fiber:** 6 g (24% of RDV)
- **Sodium:** 300 mg (13% of RDV)

53. VEGETABLE LASAGNA

 Prep time: 15 minutes   **Cooking time:** 45 minutes   **Total time:** 60 minutes   **Servings:** 1

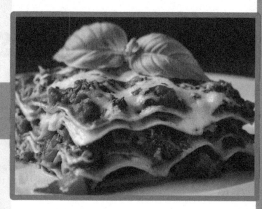

Ingredients
- **Sliced zucchini:** 1/2 cup
- **Sliced eggplant:** 1/2 cup
- **Low-fat ricotta cheese:** 1/2 cup
- **Marinara sauce:** 1 cup

American Twist:
- **Spinach:** 1/4 cup, fresh or frozen (if frozen, thawed and drained)

British Touch:
- **Sliced mushrooms:** 1/4 cup

Step-by-Step Instructions

1. **Preheat Oven:** Preheat your oven to 375°F (190°C).

2. **Prepare the Vegetables:** Lightly salt the sliced zucchini and eggplant and set aside for 10 minutes to draw out moisture. Pat dry with paper towels.

3. **Assemble the Lasagna:**

   - In a small baking dish, spread a thin layer of marinara sauce on the bottom.
   - Layer slices of zucchini and eggplant over the sauce.
   - **American Twist:** Add a layer of spinach over the zucchini and eggplant.
   - **British Touch:** Add a layer of sliced mushrooms over the zucchini and eggplant.
   - Spoon half of the ricotta cheese over the vegetables.
   - Repeat the layering process, finishing with a top layer of marinara sauce.

4. **Bake:**

   - Cover the dish with foil and bake in the preheated oven for 35 minutes.
   - Remove the foil and bake for an additional 10 minutes, or until the top is slightly browned and the vegetables are tender.

5. **Serve:** Let the lasagna cool for a few minutes before slicing to help it hold its shape when served.

Nutritional Information per Serving
- **Calories:** 350 kcal
- **Protein:** 20 g (40% of RDV)
- **Carbohydrates:** 40 g (15% of RDV)
- **Sugars:** 15 g (no daily recommended value for added sugars)
- **Fat:** 10 g (15% of RDV)
- **Saturated Fat:** 5 g (25% of RDV)
- **Fiber:** 8 g (32% of RDV)
- **Sodium:** 600 mg (26% of RDV)

54. SALMON AND SPINACH QUICHE

 Prep time: 15 minutes   **Cooking time:** 35 minutes   **Total time:** 50 minutes   **Servings:** 1

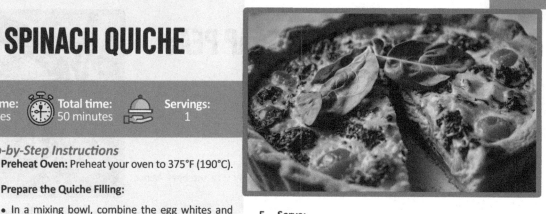

Ingredients
- **Salmon:** 1/2 cup, cooked and flaked
- **Spinach:** 1/2 cup, chopped and sautéed until wilted
- **Egg whites:** 3
- **Low-fat milk:** 1/4 cup
- **Whole wheat crust:** 1 pre-made or homemade pie crust

American Twist:
- **Dill:** 1 tbsp, chopped

British Touch:
- **Watercress:** 1/4 cup, chopped

Step-by-Step Instructions

1. **Preheat Oven:** Preheat your oven to 375°F (190°C).

2. **Prepare the Quiche Filling:**

   - In a mixing bowl, combine the egg whites and low-fat milk, whisking together until well blended.
   - Stir in the cooked salmon, sautéed spinach, and either the chopped dill **(for the American version)** or the chopped watercress **(for the British version)**, depending on your chosen twist.
   - Season the mixture with salt and pepper to taste.

3. **Assemble the Quiche:**

   - Pour the quiche filling into the whole wheat crust, spreading it evenly.
   - Ensure the salmon and greens are well distributed within the egg mixture.

4. **Bake the Quiche:**

   - Place the quiche in the preheated oven and bake for 35 minutes, or until the filling is set and the top is lightly golden.
   - Check the quiche by inserting a knife into the center; if it comes out clean, the quiche is done.

5. **Serve:**

   - Allow the quiche to cool slightly before slicing. This helps ensure clean cuts and maintains the structure of each slice.
   - Serve warm, ideally with a side salad or fresh vegetables for a complete meal.

Nutritional Information per Serving
- **Calories:** 400 kcal
- **Protein:** 28 g (56% of RDV)
- **Carbohydrates:** 30 g (11% of RDV)
- **Sugars:** 4 g (no daily recommended value for added sugars)
- **Fat:** 18 g (28% of RDV)
- **Saturated Fat:** 5 g (25% of RDV)
- **Fiber:** 5 g (20% of RDV)
- **Sodium:** 600 mg (26% of RDV)

55. CHICKEN AND BROCCOLI STIR-FRY

 Prep time: 10 minutes   **Cooking time:** 10 minutes   **Total time:** 20 minutes   **Servings:** 1

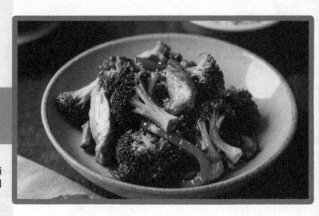

Ingredients

- **Chicken breast:** 1/2 cup, thinly sliced
- **Broccoli:** 1/2 cup, cut into florets
- **Bell peppers:** 1/4 cup, sliced
- **Soy sauce:** 1 tbsp
- **Ginger:** 1 tsp, minced

American Twist:

- **Serve over cauliflower rice:** 1/2 cup, sautéed

British Touch:

- **Cashew nuts:** 1/4 cup, toasted

Step-by-Step Instructions

1. **Prepare Ingredients:** Wash and chop the broccoli and bell peppers. Thinly slice the chicken breast and mince the ginger.

2. **Cook the Stir-Fry:**
   - Heat a small amount of oil in a wok or large frying pan over medium-high heat.
   - Add the chicken slices and stir-fry until they start to brown, about 3-4 minutes.
   - Add the minced ginger and bell peppers, stir-frying for an additional minute to release the flavors.
   - Add the broccoli and continue to stir-fry until the vegetables are tender and the chicken is fully cooked, about 3-4 more minutes.
   - Pour in the soy sauce and stir well to coat all the ingredients.

3. **American Twist:** Prepare the cauliflower rice by grating cauliflower and sautéing it in a pan with a little oil until it's tender, about 5 minutes. Serve the stir-fry over the prepared cauliflower rice as a low-carb alternative to traditional rice.

4. **British Touch:** If adding cashew nuts, toast them lightly in a dry pan until they are golden, then sprinkle over the top of the stir-fry just before serving. The cashews add a delightful crunch and nutty flavor that complements the dish.

5. **Serve:** Plate the stir-fry, either alone or over cauliflower rice, and sprinkle with toasted cashew nuts if using the British touch. Serve hot and enjoy immediately.

Nutritional Information per Serving

- **Calories:** 300 kcal
- **Protein:** 28 g (56% of RDV)
- **Carbohydrates:** 18 g (7% of RDV)
- **Sugars:** 5 g (no daily recommended value for added sugars)
- **Fat:** 12 g (18% of RDV)
- **Saturated Fat:** 2 g (10% of RDV)
- **Fiber:** 5 g (20% of RDV)
- **Sodium:** 800 mg (35% of RDV)

56. BEEF STIR-FRY WITH SNAP PEAS

 Prep time: 10 minutes   **Cooking time:** 10 minutes   **Total time:** 20 minutes   **Servings:** 1

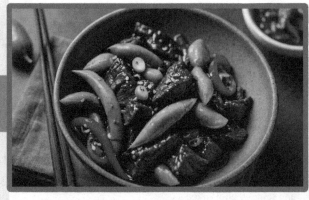

Ingredients

- **Lean beef:** 1/2 cup, thinly sliced
- **Snap peas:** 1/2 cup
- **Carrots:** 1/4 cup, julienned
- **Soy sauce:** 1 tbsp
- **Garlic:** 1 clove, minced

American Twist:

- **Sesame seeds:** 1 tbsp, toasted

British Touch:

- **Horseradish:** 1 tbsp, to serve

Step-by-Step Instructions

1. **Prepare Ingredients:** Wash and trim the snap peas. Julienned the carrots and thinly slice the beef. Mince the garlic.

2. **Cook the Stir-Fry:**
   - Heat a small amount of oil in a wok or large frying pan over medium-high heat.
   - Add the garlic and stir-fry until fragrant, about 1 minute.
   - Increase the heat to high and add the beef slices, stir-frying until they start to brown, about 3-4 minutes.
   - Add the snap peas and carrots to the pan, continuing to stir-fry until the vegetables are tender-crisp and the beef is fully cooked, about 3-4 more minutes.
   - Pour in the soy sauce and stir well to coat all the ingredients.

3. **Add Regional Twists:**
   - **American Twist:** Sprinkle toasted sesame seeds over the stir-fry before serving. The seeds add a nutty flavor and a slight crunch that enhances the texture of the dish.
   - **British Touch:** Serve the stir-fry with a side of horseradish. The pungent, spicy flavor of horseradish provides a bold contrast that complements the savory beef.

4. **Serve:** Plate the beef stir-fry, either alone or over a bed of rice or noodles. Apply the selected twist, sprinkling with sesame seeds or offering horseradish on the side, and serve immediately.

Nutritional Information per Serving

- **Calories:** 350 kcal
- **Protein:** 30 g (60% of RDV)
- **Carbohydrates:** 20 g (8% of RDV)
- **Sugars:** 5 g (no daily recommended value for added sugars)
- **Fat:** 15 g (23% of RDV)
- **Saturated Fat:** 4 g (20% of RDV)
- **Fiber:** 4 g (16% of RDV)
- **Sodium:** 900 mg (39% of RDV)

57. TOFU AND VEGETABLE STIR-FRY

 Prep time: 10 minutes   **Cooking time:** 10 minutes   **Total time:** 20 minutes **Servings:** 1

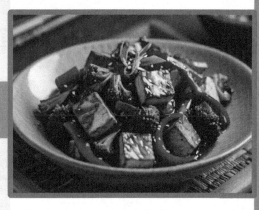

Ingredients
- **Firm tofu:** 1/2 cup, cubed and pressed
- **Mixed vegetables (such as bell peppers, broccoli, and carrots):** 1 cup
- **Teriyaki sauce:** 2 tbsps

American Twist:
- **Pineapple chunks:** 1/4 cup

British Touch:
- **Tamari (gluten-free soy sauce):** Substitute for teriyaki sauce

Step-by-Step Instructions
1. **Prepare Ingredients:** Press the tofu to remove excess moisture, then cube it. Prepare and chop the vegetables into bite-sized pieces.

2. **Cook the Tofu and Vegetables:**
   - Heat a little oil in a large pan or wok over medium-high heat.
   - Add the tofu cubes, frying until all sides are golden and crispy, about 5-7 minutes.
   - Add the mixed vegetables to the pan, stir-frying until they are just tender but still vibrant and crisp, about 3-4 minutes.

3. **Add Sauce and Twists:**
   - **Standard:** Pour the teriyaki sauce over the tofu and vegetables, stirring to coat evenly.
   - **American Twist:** Add pineapple chunks along with the teriyaki sauce. The sweetness of the pineapple enhances the savory flavors of the teriyaki sauce, adding a tropical American flair to the dish.
   - **British Touch:** If using tamari, use it in place of teriyaki sauce to add depth and a richer soy flavor, reflecting a more traditional British preference for umami profiles.

4. **Serve:** Serve the stir-fry hot, ensuring that if using the American twist, the pineapple is warm and slightly caramelized; if using the British touch, the dish has a balanced, rich soy flavor.

Nutritional Information per Serving
- **Calories:** 300 kcal
- **Protein:** 20 g (40% of RDV)
- **Carbohydrates:** 35 g (13% of RDV)
- **Sugars:** 15 g (no daily recommended value for added sugars)
- **Fat:** 10 g (15% of RDV)
- **Saturated Fat:** 1 g (5% of RDV)
- **Fiber:** 6 g (24% of RDV)
- **Sodium:** 800 mg (35% of RDV)

---

58. PORK AND ASPARAGUS STIR-FRY

 Prep time: 10 minutes   **Cooking time:** 10 minutes   **Total time:** 20 minutes   **Servings:** 1

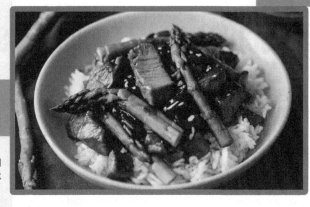

Ingredients
- **Lean pork:** 1/2 cup, thinly sliced
- **Asparagus:** 1/2 cup, trimmed and cut into 1-inch pieces
- **Mushrooms:** 1/4 cup, sliced
- **Oyster sauce:** 2 tbsps

American Twist:
- **Crushed peanuts:** 2 tbsps, for garnish

British Touch:
- **Apple cider vinegar:** 1 tbsp, mixed into the sauce

Step-by-Step Instructions
1. **Prepare Ingredients:** Trim and cut the asparagus and mushrooms. Thinly slice the lean pork to ensure quick and even cooking.

2. **Cook the Pork:** Heat a bit of oil in a wok or large frying pan over high heat. Add the pork slices and stir-fry until they start to brown, about 3-4 minutes.

3. **Add Vegetables and Sauce:**
   - Add the asparagus and mushrooms to the pan with the pork. Stir-fry for an additional 2-3 minutes until the vegetables are tender but still crisp.
   - Pour in the oyster sauce and stir to coat all the ingredients evenly.
   - **British Touch:** Add a splash of apple cider vinegar along with the oyster sauce. The vinegar adds a subtle tanginess that enhances the savory flavors of the dish.

4. **Finish and Serve:**
   - **American Twist:** Once the stir-fry is cooked, sprinkle crushed peanuts over the top before serving. The peanuts add a crunchy texture and a nutty flavor that complements the savory pork and vegetables.

5. Serve the stir-fry hot, ideally over a bed of rice or noodles to make it a complete meal.

Nutritional Information per Serving
- **Calories:** 350 kcal
- **Protein:** 25 g (50% of RDV)
- **Carbohydrates:** 15 g (6% of RDV)
- **Sugars:** 5 g (no daily recommended value for added sugars)
- **Fat:** 20 g (31% of RDV)
- **Saturated Fat:** 5 g (25% of RDV)
- **Fiber:** 3 g (12% of RDV)
- **Sodium:** 600 mg (26% of RDV)

59. LENTIL AND VEGETABLE STEW

 Prep time: 10 minutes   **Cooking time:** 30 minutes   **Total time:** 40 minutes   **Servings:** 1

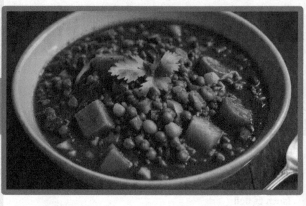

Ingredients
- **Dried lentils:** 1/2 cup (100 g)
- **Diced tomatoes:** 1 cup (240 g)
- **Zucchini, diced:** 1/2 cup (100 g)
- **Mixed herbs (thyme, rosemary, parsley), chopped:** 1 tbsp
- **Vegetable broth:** 2 cups (480 ml)
- **Onion, chopped:** 1/4 cup (40 g)
- **Garlic, minced:** 1 clove
- **Olive oil:** 1 tsp
- **Salt and pepper:** to taste

American Touch:
- **Pesto:** 1 tbsp

British Touch:
- **Stout beer:** 1 tbsp

Step-by-Step Instructions
1. **Sauté Aromatics:** In a large pot, heat the olive oil over medium heat. Add the chopped onion and minced garlic, sautéing until the onions become translucent, about 3-4 minutes.
2. **Cook Vegetables:** Add the diced zucchini to the pot and sauté for another 5 minutes, until slightly softened.
3. **Simmer Lentils:** Stir in the dried lentils, diced tomatoes, and vegetable broth. Bring the mixture to a boil, then reduce the heat to low and let it simmer, covered, for about 20 minutes or until the lentils are tender.

   • **American Touch:** Stir in a tbsp of pesto into the stew just before removing it from heat, for a rich and herby flavor enhancement.
   • **British Touch:** Add a tbsp of stout beer during the last 5 minutes of simmering to infuse a deep, malty undertone to the stew.
4. **Season:** Add the chopped herbs, and season with salt and pepper to taste. Adjust the seasoning and consistency of the stew according to your preferences.
5. **Serve:** Serve the stew hot, perfect for a comforting and hearty meal.

Tips and Variations
- **Extra Vegetables:** Feel free to add carrots, celery, or bell peppers for more texture and nutrition.
- **Vegan Protein Boost:** Include chunks of tofu or a scoop of cooked quinoa for added protein.

Storage and Serving Suggestions
- **Storage:** This stew can be stored in the refrigerator for up to 3 days or frozen for up to a month. Reheat gently on the stove or in a microwave.

Nutritional Information per Serving
- **Calories:** 325 kcal - **Protein:** 18 g (36% of RDV)
- **Carbohydrates:** 50 g (17%) - **Sugars:** 10 g
- **Fat:** 7 g (11%) - **Saturated Fat:** 1 g (5%)
- **Fiber:** 15 g (60%) - **Sodium:** 300 mg (13%)

60. QUINOA STUFFED PEPPERS

 Prep time: 15 minutes   **Cooking time:** 25 minutes   **Total time:** 40 minutes   **Servings:** 1

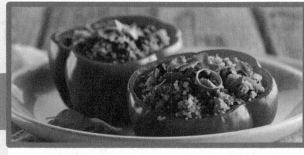

Ingredients
- **Quinoa:** 1/4 cup (45 g)
- **Black beans, drained and rinsed:** 1/4 cup (40 g)
- **Corn, fresh or frozen:** 1/4 cup (40 g)
- **Tomatoes, diced:** 1/4 cup (40 g)
- **Bell peppers, any color:** 2 halves
- **Onion, finely chopped:** 2 tbsps
- **Garlic, minced:** 1 clove
- **Olive oil:** 1 tsp
- **Cumin powder:** 1/2 tsp
- **Chili powder:** 1/4 tsp
- **Salt and pepper:** to taste

American Touch:
- **Avocado, sliced:** 1/4 (50 g)

British Touch:
- **Mint yogurt:** 2 tbsps

Step-by-Step Instructions
1. **Preheat Oven and Prepare Quinoa:** Preheat your oven to 375°F (190°C). Cook quinoa according to package instructions, typically simmering in double the amount of water for about 15 minutes until tender and water is absorbed.
2. **Prepare Vegetable Mixture:** While the quinoa cooks, heat olive oil in a skillet over medium heat. Add the chopped onion and minced garlic, sautéing until onions are translucent. Stir in the black beans, corn, and tomatoes. Season with cumin, chili powder, salt, and pepper. Cook for another 5 minutes until the mixture is heated through.
3. **Combine with Quinoa:** Mix the cooked quinoa into the skillet with the vegetable mixture, ensuring everything is well combined.
4. **Stuff Peppers:** Cut the bell peppers in half lengthwise, removing the seeds. Place the pepper halves in a baking dish and fill each with the quinoa mixture.
5. **Bake:** Place the stuffed peppers in the preheated oven and bake for about 20 minutes, or until the peppers are tender and the filling is hot.

   • **American Touch:** Top the baked stuffed peppers with avocado slices just before serving for a creamy texture and a boost of healthy fats.
   • **British Touch:** Drizzle mint yogurt over the stuffed peppers for a refreshing contrast and a hint of coolness.
6. **Serve:** Enjoy the colorful and nutritious stuffed peppers warm.

Tips and Variations
- **Cheese Option:** For extra flavor, sprinkle some grated cheddar or feta cheese over the peppers before baking.
- **Spice It Up:** Add a pinch of red pepper flakes to the quinoa mixture for extra heat if desired.

Storage and Serving Suggestions
- **Storage:** These stuffed peppers can be refrigerated for up to 3 days. Reheat in the microwave or oven until warmed throughout.
- **Make Ahead:** Prepare the quinoa and vegetable mixture in advance and store in the fridge for easy assembly and baking later.

Nutritional Information per Serving
- **Calories:** 350 kcal - **Protein:** 10 g (20% of RDV)
- **Carbohydrates:** 45 g (15%) - **Sugars:** 6 g
- **Fat:** 15 g (23%) - **Saturated Fat:** 2 g (10%)
- **Fiber:** 10 g (40%) - **Sodium:** 250 mg (10.4%)

61. VEGETABLE PAELLA

 Prep time: 10 minutes **Cooking time:** 25 minutes **Total time:** 35 minutes **Servings:** 1

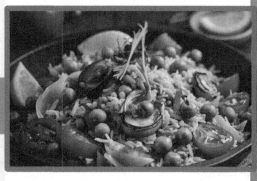

Ingredients

- **Saffron rice:** 1/2 cup (90 g) uncooked
- **Artichokes, quartered:** 1/4 cup (30 g)
- **Bell peppers, colors, diced:** 1/4 cup (40g)
- **Peas, fresh or frozen:** 1/4 cup (40 g)
- **Tomatoes, diced:** 1/4 cup (40 g)
- **Onion, finely chopped:** 2 tbsps
- **Garlic, minced:** 1 clove
- **Vegetable broth:** 1 cup (240 ml)
- **Olive oil:** 1 tsp
- **Saffron threads:** a pinch
- **Salt and pepper:** to taste

American Touch:
- **Roasted red peppers, sliced:** 1/4 cup (40 g)

British Touch:
- **Smoked paprika:** 1/2 tsp

Step-by-Step Instructions

1. **Prepare Saffron Rice:** In a small bowl, soak the saffron threads in a tbsp of warm water for about 5 minutes to release the color and flavor.
2. **Cook the Paella:** Heat the olive oil in a shallow pan or skillet over medium heat. Add the chopped onion and minced garlic, cooking until the onion is translucent.
3. **Add Vegetables:** Stir in the bell peppers, artichokes, peas, and diced tomatoes. Cook for about 5 minutes, stirring occasionally.
4. **Add Rice and Broth:** Mix in the saffron along with its soaking liquid and the uncooked rice. Pour in the vegetable broth and bring to a simmer. Season with salt and pepper, and add the smoked paprika for the British touch.
5. **Simmer:** Reduce the heat to low, cover, and let the paella cook for about 18-20 minutes, or until the rice is tender and the liquid is absorbed. Avoid stirring too much as paella is best when it forms a slight crust on the bottom.

   • **American Touch:** Stir in the roasted red peppers about halfway through the cooking time to incorporate their sweet, smoky flavor into the dish.

6. **Finish and Serve:** Once the rice is cooked and the vegetables are tender, remove from heat. Let it sit covered for a few minutes before serving to allow the flavors to meld.

7. **Serve:** Dish out the colorful vegetable paella onto a plate, garnishing with fresh herbs if desired, and enjoy the vibrant flavors.

Tips and Variations
- **Protein Boost:** Add chickpeas or a plant-based sausage sliced into rounds for extra protein.
- **More Heat:** Include a dash of cayenne pepper if you prefer a spicier dish.

Storage and Serving Suggestions
- **Storage:** Refrigerate any leftovers in an airtight container for up to 2 days. Reheat gently, adding a little water if the rice has dried out.
- **Make Ahead:** Chop all the vegetables in advance and store them in the fridge for a quick assembly when you're ready to cook.

Nutritional Information per Serving
- **Calories:** 380 kcal - **Protein:** 8 g (16% of RDV)
- **Carbohydrates:** 65 g (22%) - **Sugars:** 8 g
- **Fat:** 9 g (14%) - **Saturated Fat:** 1.5 g (7.5%)
- **Fiber:** 9 g (36%) - **Sodium:** 600 mg (25%)

62. VEGETABLE STICKS WITH HUMMUS

 Prep time: 10 minutes **Cooking time:** Not Expected **Total time:** 10 minutes **Servings:** 1

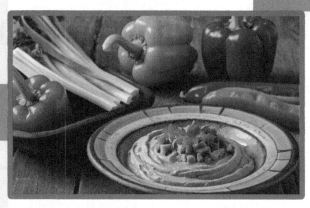

Ingredients

- **Carrots, peeled and cut into sticks:** 1 medium (60 g)
- **Celery, cut into sticks:** 1 stalk (40 g)
- **Bell peppers, assorted colors, cut into sticks:** 1/2 pepper (60 g)
- **Chickpeas, drained and rinsed:** 1/2 cup (120 g)
- **Lemon juice:** 1 tbsp
- **Tahini (sesame paste):** 1 tbsp
- **Garlic, minced:** 1 clove
- **Ground cumin:** 1/2 tsp
- **Salt:** to taste
- **Water:** as needed for consistency

American Touch:
- **Smoked paprika:** 1/2tsp

British Touch:
- **Onion powder:** 1/2 tsp

Step-by-Step Instructions

1. **Prepare the Hummus:** In a food processor or blender, combine the chickpeas, lemon juice, tahini, minced garlic, ground cumin, salt, and a few tbsps of water. Blend until smooth. If the hummus is too thick, gradually add more water until you reach the desired consistency.
2. **Add Flavors:**

   • **American Twist:** Mix in the smoked paprika with the hummus blend for a smoky flavor.
   • **British Touch:** Stir in the onion powder to enhance the hummus with a savory onion taste.

3. **Prepare Vegetable Sticks:** Wash and cut the carrots, celery, and bell peppers into stick shapes suitable for dipping.
4. **Serve:** Arrange the vegetable sticks neatly on a plate alongside the bowl of flavored hummus.
5. **Enjoy:** Dip the vegetable sticks into the hummus and savor the fresh, crisp textures paired with the creamy, spiced hummus.

Tips and Variations
- **Extra Creaminess:** Add a spoonful of Greek yogurt to the hummus for extra creaminess without added oil.
- **Spice It Up:** For an extra kick, sprinkle a little chili powder or cayenne pepper into the hummus mix.

Storage and Serving Suggestions
- **Storage:** The hummus can be stored in the refrigerator in an airtight container for up to 5 days. The vegetable sticks should be prepared fresh, though they can be cut and stored in water in the refrigerator for up to 2 days.
- **Serving Suggestion:** This dish makes an excellent snack or appetizer for gatherings, providing a healthy option that is both flavorful and satisfying.

Nutritional Information per Serving
- **Calories:** 265 kcal - **Protein:** 9 g (18% of RDV)
- **Carbohydrates:** 30 g (10%) - **Sugars:** 6 g
- **Fat:** 14 g (22%) - **Saturated Fat:** 2 g (10%)
- **Fiber:** 8 g (32%) - **Sodium:** 300 mg (12.5%)

63. BAKED KALE CHIPS

 Prep time: 5 minutes 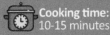 **Cooking time:** 10-15 minutes 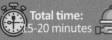 **Total time:** 15-20 minutes **Servings:** 1

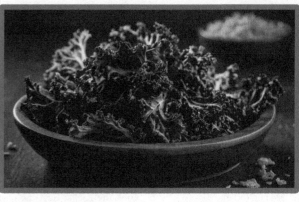

Ingredients
- Kale, stems removed and leaves torn into bite-sized pieces: 1 large bunch (about 200 g)
- Olive oil spray
- Sea salt: to taste

American Touch:
- Apple cider vinegar powder: 1/2 tsp

British Touch:
- Nutritional yeast: 1 tbsp

Step-by-Step Instructions
1. **Preheat Oven and Prepare Kale:** Preheat your oven to 350°F (175°C). Wash the kale leaves thoroughly and dry them completely using a salad spinner or patting them dry with towels. It's important that the kale is very dry to ensure it becomes crispy.
2. **Season the Kale:** Spread the kale pieces on a baking sheet lined with parchment paper. Lightly spray the kale with olive oil and then sprinkle with sea salt.
   - **American Twist:** Dust the kale with apple cider vinegar powder for a tangy flavor.
   - **British Touch:** Sprinkle nutritional yeast over the kale for a cheesy flavor and added vitamins.
3. **Bake:** Place the kale in the oven and bake for 10-15 minutes, or until the edges are brown but not burnt. The baking time may vary depending on the oven, so keep a close eye on the kale to prevent overcooking.
4. **Cool and Serve:** Remove the kale chips from the oven and let them cool on the baking sheet for a few minutes to crisp up further.
5. **Enjoy:** Serve the crispy kale chips immediately for the best texture, or store them in an airtight container once completely cooled.

Tips and Variations
- **Flavor Variants:** Experiment with different seasonings like chili powder, garlic powder, or smoked paprika for variety.
- **Even Cooking:** Make sure the kale pieces are in a single layer on the baking sheet to ensure they cook evenly.

Storage and Serving Suggestions
- **Storage:** Kale chips are best enjoyed fresh but can be stored in an airtight container for up to 2 days. Note that they might lose some of their crispiness over time.
- **Portable Snack:** Perfect for on-the-go snacking or as a healthy alternative to traditional chips at gatherings.

Nutritional Information per Serving
- **Calories:** 150 kcal - **Protein:** 5 g (10% of RDV)
- **Carbohydrates:** 10 g (3%) - **Sugars:** 0 g
- **Fat:** 10 g (15%) - **Saturated Fat:** 1.5 g (7.5%)
- **Fiber:** 2 g (8%) - **Sodium:** 200 mg (8.3%)

64. APPLE SLICES WITH ALMOND BUTTER

 Prep time: 5 minutes **Cooking time:** Not Expected **Total time:** 5 minutes **Servings:** 1

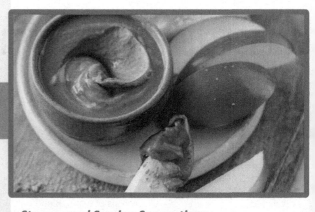

Ingredients
- Apple, medium-sized, cored and sliced: 1 (about 200 g)
- Natural almond butter: 2 tbsps (30 g)

American Touch:
- Cinnamon: 1/4 tsp

British Touch:
- Ground ginger: 1/4 tsp

Step-by-Step Instructions
1. **Prepare Apple:** Wash the apple thoroughly. Core and slice it into even pieces for easy eating and dipping.
2. **Enhance Almond Butter:**
   - **American Twist:** Stir cinnamon into the almond butter for a warm, spicy flavor that complements the sweetness of the apple.
   - **British Touch:** Mix ground ginger into the almond butter, adding a slightly sharp and zesty flavor that contrasts nicely with the apple.
3. **Serve:** Place the sliced apple on a plate with the enhanced almond butter on the side for dipping.
4. **Enjoy:** Dip apple slices into the almond butter and enjoy the delightful combination of flavors.

Tips and Variations
- **Variety of Apples:** Experiment with different types of apples like Granny Smith for tartness or Honeycrisp for extra sweetness.
- **Extra Crunch:** Sprinkle a few chopped almonds on top of the almond butter for added texture and flavor.
- **Nut Butter Options:** Feel free to substitute peanut butter or cashew butter if preferred.

Storage and Serving Suggestions
- **Immediate Consumption:** This snack is best enjoyed immediately after preparation to maintain the freshness and crispness of the apples.
- **Prep Ahead:** If preparing in advance, brush the apple slices with a little lemon juice to prevent browning.

Nutritional Information per Serving
- **Calories:** 280 kcal
- **Protein:** 6 g (12% of RDV)
- **Carbohydrates:** 34 g (11%)
- **Sugars:** 23 g
- **Fat:** 16 g (24%)
- **Saturated Fat:** 1.5 g (7.5%)
- **Fiber:** 6 g (24%)
- **Sodium:** 5 mg (0.2%)

65. GREEK YOGURT WITH BERRIES

 Prep time: 5 minutes **Cooking time:** Not Expected **Total time:** 5 minutes **Servings:** 1

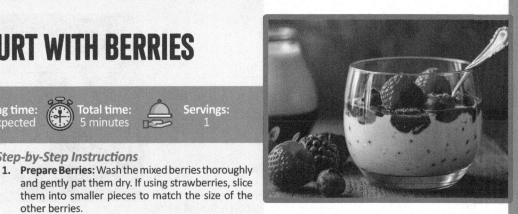

Ingredients
- **Non-fat Greek yogurt:** 1 cup (245 g)
- **Mixed berries (strawberries, blueberries, raspberries, blackberries):** 1/2 cup (70 g)

American Touch:
- **Sugar-free maple syrup:** 1 tbsp (15 ml)

British Touch:
- **Sugar-free blackcurrant preserve:** 1 tbsp (15 ml)

Step-by-Step Instructions
1. **Prepare Berries:** Wash the mixed berries thoroughly and gently pat them dry. If using strawberries, slice them into smaller pieces to match the size of the other berries.

2. **Assemble the Yogurt Bowl:** Spoon the Greek yogurt into a serving bowl. Top with the prepared mixed berries.

3. **Add Flavors:**
   - **American Twist:** Drizzle sugar-free maple syrup over the yogurt and berries for a sweet, aromatic flavor.
   - **British Touch:** Dollop sugar-free blackcurrant preserve on top of the yogurt, offering a tangy contrast to the creamy yogurt and sweet berries.

4. **Serve:** Gently mix at the table to swirl the maple syrup and blackcurrant preserve into the yogurt before eating, or enjoy the distinct layers of flavors in each spoonful.

Tips and Variations
- **Extra Texture:** Add a sprinkle of toasted nuts or seeds for a crunchy texture.

- **Protein Boost:** Stir a scoop of protein powder into the yogurt before adding the berries for an added protein kick.

Storage and Serving Suggestions
- **Best Served Fresh:** This dish is best enjoyed immediately after preparation to maintain the freshness of the berries and the creaminess of the yogurt.
- **Prep in Advance:** If preparing for later, store the yogurt and berries separately in the refrigerator and assemble just before serving to prevent the berries from becoming too soft.

Nutritional Information per Serving
- **Calories:** 180 kcal - **Protein:** 20 g (40% of RDV)
- **Carbohydrates:** 25 g (8%) - **Sugars:** 12 g
- **Fat:** 0 g (0%) - **Saturated Fat:** 0 g (0%)
- **Fiber:** 3 g (12%) - **Sodium:** 65 mg (2.7%)

---

66. CHIA SEED PUDDING

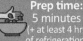 **Prep time:** 5 minutes (+ at least 4 hrs of refrigeration) **Cooking time:** Not Expected **Total time:** 4 hours 5 minutes **Servings:** 1

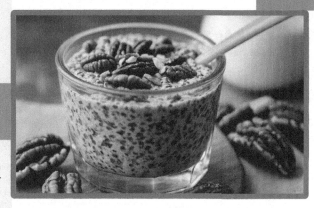

Ingredients
- **Chia seeds:** 3 tbsps (45 g)
- **Unsweetened almond milk:** 1 cup (240 ml)
- **Vanilla extract:** 1 tsp (5 ml)

American Touch:
- **Sugar-free pecans, chopped:** 2 tbsps (15 g)

British Touch:
- **Stewed rhubarb:** 1/4 cup (60 g)

Step-by-Step Instructions
1. **Mix Ingredients:** In a mixing bowl, combine the chia seeds, unsweetened almond milk, and vanilla extract. Stir thoroughly to mix well and ensure there are no clumps.

2. **Refrigerate:** Cover the bowl with a lid or plastic wrap and refrigerate for at least 4 hours, preferably overnight, to allow the chia seeds to absorb the liquid and form a gel-like pudding texture.

3. **Prepare Toppings:**
   - **American Twist:** Toast the chopped pecans in a dry skillet over medium heat for about 3-5 minutes until they are golden and fragrant. Set aside to cool.
   - **British Touch:** Prepare the stewed rhubarb by simmering chopped rhubarb with a bit of water and a sweetener of choice (like stevia or erythritol) until soft and broken down, about 10 minutes. Let cool.

4. **Assemble:** Once the chia pudding has set, stir it well to break up any lumps. Spoon the pudding into a serving dish.

5. **Add Toppings:** Sprinkle the toasted pecans over the pudding for a crunchy texture and nutty flavor. Top with a layer of stewed rhubarb for a tangy contrast to the sweet and creamy pudding.

6. **Serve:** Enjoy this nutritious and satisfying chia seed pudding as a breakfast, dessert, or snack.

Tips and Variations
- **Flavor Enhancements:** Add a pinch of cinnamon or nutmeg to the pudding mix for extra flavor.
- **Alternative Milks:** Feel free to use other types of milk like coconut milk or oat milk for different flavors and textures.

Storage and Serving Suggestions
- **Storage:** Chia pudding can be stored in the refrigerator for up to 5 days. It's perfect for preparing in advance for quick and easy meals throughout the week.
- **Serving Cold:** This dish is best served cold, providing a refreshing treat especially in warm weather.

Nutritional Information per Serving
- **Calories:** 290 kcal - **Protein:** 6 g (12% of RDV)
- **Carbohydrates:** 25 g (8%) - **Sugars:** 3 g
- **Fat:** 18 g (28%) - **Saturated Fat:** 1.5 g (7.5%)
- **Fiber:** 10 g (40%) - **Sodium:** 180 mg (7.5%)

67. HARD-BOILED EGGS

 Prep time: 2 minutes   **Cooking time:** 10 minutes   **Total time:** 12 minutes   **Servings:** 1

Ingredients
- **Eggs:** 2 large

American Touch:
- **Chili powder:** 1/4 tsp

British Touch:
- **Branston pickle:** 1 tbsp

Step-by-Step Instructions
1. **Cook the Eggs:** Place the eggs in a saucepan and cover them with cold water by 1 inch. Bring the water to a boil over medium-high heat. Once boiling, cover the pan with a lid, turn off the heat, and let the eggs sit in the hot water for 9-10 minutes for firm yet creamy yolks.

2. **Cool the Eggs:** After cooking, transfer the eggs to a bowl of ice water or run them under cold tap water for a few minutes to stop the cooking process. This also makes peeling easier.

3. **Peel the Eggs:** Gently crack the shells and peel them off the eggs. Rinse the eggs under water to remove any small shell pieces.

4. **Add Flavors:**
   - **American Twist:** Sprinkle chili powder over the eggs for a spicy kick.
   - **British Touch:** Serve the eggs with a side of Branston pickle for a tangy and slightly sweet complement.

5. **Serve:** Enjoy the hard-boiled eggs whole or sliced in half, seasoned with chili powder and accompanied by Branston pickle on the side.

Tips and Variations
- **Additional Toppings:** Add a pinch of salt, a dash of black pepper, or paprika for extra flavor.
- **Serving Suggestions:** These eggs can be a great addition to salads, sandwiches, or simply enjoyed on their own as a protein-rich snack.

Storage and Serving Suggestions
- **Storage:** Hard-boiled eggs can be stored in the refrigerator with their shells on for up to a week. If peeled, store them in an airtight container or tightly wrapped in plastic wrap to prevent drying out.
- **Quick Snack:** Hard-boiled eggs are an excellent grab-and-go snack, making them a convenient and healthy option for busy days.

Nutritional Information per Serving
- **Calories:** 140 kcal - **Protein:** 12 g (24% of RDV)
- **Carbohydrates:** 1 g (<1%) - **Sugars:** 0 g
- **Fat:** 10 g (15%) - **Saturated Fat:** 3 g (15%)
- **Fiber:** 0 g (0%) - **Sodium:** 120 mg (5%)

68. EDAMAME PODS

 Prep time: 2 minutes   **Cooking time:** 5 minutes   **Total time:** 7 minutes   **Servings:** 1

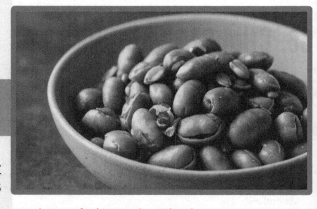

Ingredients
- **Edamame (fresh or frozen):** 1 cup (150 g)
- **Sea salt:** to taste

American Touch:
- **Garlic powder:** 1/2 tsp
- **Lime:** 1, cut into wedges

British Touch:
- **Malt vinegar powder:** 1/2 tsp

Step-by-Step Instructions
1. **Cook the Edamame:** If using frozen edamame, there's no need to thaw them. Bring a pot of water to a boil. Add the edamame and cook for about 5 minutes, or until they are tender and bright green.

2. **Drain and Season:** Drain the edamame in a colander and immediately sprinkle with sea salt.

3. **Add Flavors:**
   - **American Twist:** Sprinkle garlic powder over the hot edamame. Serve with lime wedges on the side, allowing the option to squeeze fresh lime juice over the pods before eating for a zesty, flavorful kick.
   - **British Touch:** Dust the pods with malt vinegar powder, giving them a tangy and distinctive British pub-snack flavor.

4. **Serve:** Enjoy the edamame hot as a nutritious and satisfying snack.

Tips and Variations
- **Enhance Flavor:** Experiment with other spices such as smoked paprika or chili flakes for additional flavor profiles.
- **Serve Cold:** These can also be enjoyed cold, making them a refreshing snack on a hot day.

Storage and Serving Suggestions
- **Storage:** Leftover edamame can be stored in the refrigerator for up to three days. Reheat in the microwave or enjoy cold.
- **Great for Gatherings:** Edamame pods make a great appetizer or snack for parties and gatherings, offering a healthful option that's also fun to eat.

Nutritional Information per Serving
- **Calories:** 190 kcal
- **Protein:** 17 g (34% of RDV)
- **Carbohydrates:** 14 g (5%)
- **Sugars:** 3 g
- **Fat:** 8 g (12%)
- **Saturated Fat:** 1 g (5%)
- **Fiber:** 8 g (32%)
- **Sodium:** 300 mg (13%)

69. COTTAGE CHEESE WITH PINEAPPLE

 Prep time: 5 minutes **Cooking time:** Not Expected **Total time:** 5 minutes **Servings:** 1

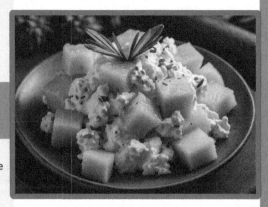

Ingredients
- **Low-fat cottage cheese:** 1 cup (225 g)
- **Diced pineapple:** 1/2 cup (75 g)

American Touch:
- **Cinnamon:** 1/4 tsp

British Touch:
- **Minced mint:** 1 tbsp

Step-by-Step Instructions
1. **Prepare Ingredients:** In a serving bowl, combine the low-fat cottage cheese with the diced pineapple.

2. **Add Flavors:**

   - **American Twist:** Sprinkle cinnamon over the cottage cheese and pineapple mixture for a warm, spicy flavor that complements the sweetness of the pineapple.
   - **British Touch:** Mix in minced mint with the cottage cheese and pineapple, providing a fresh, aromatic contrast to the dish.

3. **Serve:** Stir everything together gently until well combined, and enjoy this refreshing and healthful dish.

Tips and Variations
- **Enhance Texture:** For added crunch, sprinkle some chopped nuts or seeds over the top.
- **Protein Boost:** For an extra protein kick, mix a scoop of protein powder into the cottage cheese before adding the other ingredients.

Storage and Serving Suggestions
- **Immediate Consumption:** This dish is best enjoyed fresh due to the fresh ingredients used.
- **Prep Ahead:** You can mix the cottage cheese and cinnamon or mint ahead of time and store it in the fridge, then add the fresh pineapple just before serving.

Nutritional Information per Serving
- **Calories:** 200 kcal
- **Protein:** 20 g (40% of RDV)
- **Carbohydrates:** 20 g (7%)
- **Sugars:** 15 g
- **Fat:** 2 g (3%)
- **Saturated Fat:** 1 g (5%)
- **Fiber:** 1 g (4%)
- **Sodium:** 500 mg (21.7%)

70. ROASTED CHICKPEAS

 Prep time: 10 minutes **Cooking time:** 30-40 minutes 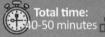 **Total time:** 40-50 minutes **Servings:** 1

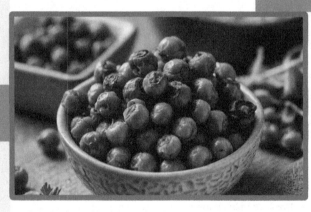

Ingredients
- **Chickpeas, canned, drained and rinsed:** 1 cup (240 g)
- **Olive oil:** 1 tbsp (15 ml)
- **Cumin:** 1/2 tsp
- **Paprika:** 1/2 tsp

American Touch: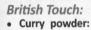
- **Ranch flavoring:** 1 tsp

British Touch:
- **Curry powder:** 1 tsp

Step-by-Step Instructions
1. **Preheat Oven and Prepare Chickpeas:** Preheat your oven to 400°F (200°C). After rinsing the chickpeas, pat them dry with paper towels. It's important to remove as much moisture as possible to achieve a crispy texture.
2. **Season the Chickpeas:** Place the chickpeas in a bowl. Add olive oil, cumin, and paprika, tossing well to ensure all chickpeas are evenly coated.
3. **Add Flavors:**

   - **American Twist:** Sprinkle the ranch flavoring over the chickpeas for a tangy, herby taste.
   - **British Touch:** Add curry powder to the chickpeas for a spicy, aromatic kick.
4. **Bake:** Spread the chickpeas in a single layer on a baking sheet lined with parchment paper. Roast in the preheated oven for 30-40 minutes, stirring every 10 minutes to ensure even cooking and crispiness.
5. **Cool and Serve:** Remove the chickpeas from the oven and let them cool on the baking sheet for a few minutes to further crisp up.
6. **Enjoy:** Serve the roasted chickpeas as a snack or as a crunchy addition to salads or soups.

Tips and Variations
- **Additional Spices:** Feel free to experiment with other spices such as garlic powder, onion powder, or chili powder for different flavors.
- **Cooking Time:** Adjust the cooking time depending on your oven and desired crispiness. Watch the chickpeas carefully towards the end to prevent burning.

Storage and Serving Suggestions
- **Storage:** Store the roasted chickpeas in an airtight container at room temperature. They are best eaten within a day or two as they lose their crispiness over time.
- **Portable Snack:** These make an excellent portable snack for outings or work, providing a healthy, protein-rich alternative to traditional snack foods.

Nutritional Information per Serving
- **Calories:** 365 kcal - **Protein:** 12 g (24% of RDV)
- **Carbohydrates:** 45 g (15%) - **Sugars:** 8 g
- **Fat:** 18 g (28%) - **Saturated Fat:** 2.5 g (12.5%)
- **Fiber:** 12 g (48%) - **Sodium:** 300 mg (13%)

71. ZUCCHINI CHIPS

 Prep time: 10 minutes   **Cooking time:** 20-30 minutes 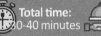 **Total time:** 30-40 minutes **Servings:** 1

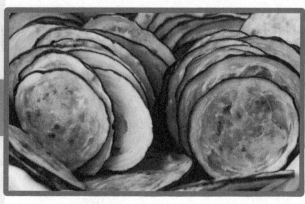

Ingredients
- Zucchini, medium-sized, thinly sliced: 1 (about 200 g)
- Olive oil spray
- Salt: to taste

American Touch:
- Ranch seasoning: 1 tsp

British Touch:
- Vinegar powder: 1 tsp

Step-by-Step Instructions
1. **Preheat Oven and Prepare Zucchini:** Preheat your oven to 425°F (220°C). Using a mandoline slicer or a very sharp knife, slice the zucchini into thin, even slices to ensure they cook evenly.

2. **Season the Zucchini:** Arrange the zucchini slices in a single layer on a baking sheet lined with parchment paper. Lightly spray with olive oil and sprinkle with salt.
   - **American Twist:** Sprinkle ranch seasoning over the zucchini slices for a tangy, herby flavor.
   - **British Touch:** Dust with vinegar powder to give the chips a sharp, tangy taste reminiscent of salt and vinegar chips.

3. **Bake:** Place the baking sheet in the preheated oven and bake for 20-30 minutes, or until the zucchini chips are golden and crisp. Make sure to turn the slices halfway through the baking time to ensure even crisping.

4. **Cool and Serve:** Remove the chips from the oven and let them cool on the baking sheet for a few minutes to further crisp up.

5. **Enjoy:** Serve the zucchini chips as a light, crunchy snack.

Tips and Variations
- **Watch Carefully:** Keep a close eye on the chips, especially towards the end of baking, as they can easily go from crisp to burnt.
- **Additional Flavors:** Experiment with other seasoning mixes such as garlic powder, smoked paprika, or chili flakes to vary the flavors.

Storage and Serving Suggestions
- **Best Served Fresh:** These chips are best enjoyed immediately after cooking while they are still crispy.
- **Storage:** If you have leftovers, store them in an airtight container for up to 1 day, though they may lose some crispness.

Nutritional Information per Serving
- **Calories:** 120 kcal - **Protein:** 3 g (6% of RDV)
- **Carbohydrates:** 10 g (3%) - **Sugars:** 7 g
- **Fat:** 8 g (12%) - **Saturated Fat:** 1 g (5%)
- **Fiber:** 3 g (12%) - **Sodium:** 200 mg (8.3%)

72. PROTEIN SMOOTHIE

 Prep time: 5 minutes   **Cooking time:** Not Expected   **Total time:** 5 minutes   **Servings:** 1

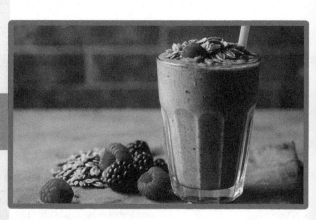

Ingredients
- **Protein powder:** 1 scoop (approximately 30 g)
- **Unsweetened almond milk:** 1 cup (240 ml)
- **Frozen berries (such as blueberries, strawberries, and raspberries):** 1/2 cup (70 g)

American Twist:
- **Peanut butter:** 1 tbsp (15 g)

British Touch:
- **Rolled oats:** 2 tbsps (20 g)

Step-by-Step Instructions
1. **Combine Ingredients:** In a blender, add the protein powder, unsweetened almond milk, frozen berries, peanut butter, and rolled oats.

2. **Blend:** Blend on high speed until the mixture is smooth and creamy. Ensure all ingredients are thoroughly combined and the oats have been fully integrated, creating a smooth texture.

3. **Adjust Consistency:** If the smoothie is too thick, add a little more almond milk to achieve the desired consistency. If it's too thin, add more frozen berries or a few ice cubes and blend again.

4. **Serve:** Pour the smoothie into a large glass or a shaker bottle if you're on the go.

5. **Enjoy:** Drink immediately to enjoy the best flavor and nutritional benefits.

Tips and Variations
- **Protein Options:** Feel free to use different types of protein powder, such as whey, soy, or pea protein, to suit dietary preferences or needs.
- **Flavor Boost:** Add a pinch of vanilla extract or cinnamon for additional flavor layers.

Storage and Serving Suggestions
- **Immediate Consumption:** This smoothie is best enjoyed immediately after blending to maximize the freshness and nutritional benefits.
- **Prep Ahead:** You can prepare the dry ingredients in a blender container the night before, store in the refrigerator, and just blend with almond milk and peanut butter in the morning for a quick breakfast.

Nutritional Information per Serving
- **Calories:** 320 kcal - **Protein:** 28 g (56% of RDV)
- **Carbohydrates:** 26 g (9%) - **Sugars:** 12 g | Fat: 12 g (18%)
- **Saturated Fat:** 2 g (10%) - **Fiber:** 5 g (20%)
- **Sodium:** 250 mg (10.4%)

DESSERTS

73. CHIA PUDDING WITH MIXED BERRIES

 Prep time: least 4 hours of **Total time:** **Servings:**
5 minutes (+ at refrigeration) hours 5 minutes 1

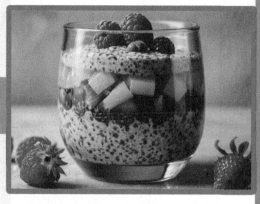

Ingredients

- **Chia seeds:** 3 tbsps (45 g)
- **Unsweetened almond milk:** 1 cup (240 ml)
- **Mixed berries (such as strawberries, blueberries, raspberries):** 1/2 cup (70 g)

American Twist:
- **Vanilla extract:** 1/2 tsp

British Touch:
- **Sugar-free lemon curd:** 2 tbsps (30 ml)

Step-by-Step Instructions

1. **Mix Ingredients:** In a bowl, combine the chia seeds and unsweetened almond milk. Stir thoroughly to prevent clumping.
2. **Flavor Addition:**
   - **American Twist:** Add the vanilla extract to the chia seed mixture for a sweet and aromatic flavor.
   - **British twist:** add sugar-free lemon curd to the mixture.
3. **Refrigerate:** Cover the bowl with a lid or plastic wrap and refrigerate for at least 4 hours, preferably overnight, to allow the chia seeds to absorb the almond milk and swell, forming a gel-like consistency.
4. **Prepare Berries:** Wash and slice any larger berries if necessary, ensuring all are ready to layer or mix into the pudding.
5. **Assemble Pudding:** Layer half of the prepared chia pudding at the bottom of a serving glass.
   - Add a layer of mixed berries.
   - Spoon a layer of sugar-free lemon curd over the berries for the British touch.
   - Top with the remaining chia pudding.
   - Finish with another layer of mixed berries.
6. **Serve:** Enjoy this delicious and nutritious dessert that's perfect for a healthy treat or a light breakfast.

Tips and Variations
- **Enhance Nutrients:** Add a sprinkle of ground flaxseeds or hemp seeds for extra fiber and omega-3 fatty acids.
- **Additional Toppings:** Consider garnishing with nuts or coconut flakes for added texture and flavor.

Storage and Serving Suggestions
- **Storage:** Chia pudding can be stored in the refrigerator for up to 5 days, making it a great make-ahead option.
- **Serving Cold:** Serve chilled to enjoy the most refreshing taste and texture.

Nutritional Information per Serving
- **Calories:** 300 kcal - **Protein:** 10 g (20% of RDV)
- **Carbohydrates:** 35 g (12%) - **Sugars:** 10 g
- **Fat:** 15 g (23%) - **Saturated Fat:** 1.5 g (7.5%)
- **Fiber:** 15 g (60%) - **Sodium:** 180 mg (7.8%)

74. BAKED APPLE SLICES

 Prep time: **Cooking time:** **Total time:** **Servings:**
5 minutes 15-20 minutes 20-25 minutes 1

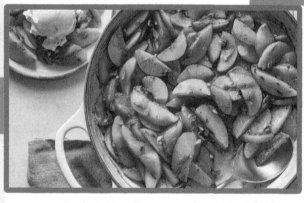

Ingredients

- **Apple, large, cored and sliced into rounds or wedges:** 1 (about 200 g)
- **Cinnamon:** 1/2 tsp
- **Nutmeg:** 1/4 tsp

American Twist:
- **Sugar-free whipped cream:** for serving

British Touch:
- **Sugar-free custard powder:** 1 tbsp

Step-by-Step Instructions

1. **Preheat Oven and Prepare Apples:** Preheat your oven to 375°F (190°C). Core and slice the apple into even rounds or wedges, depending on your preference.
2. **Season the Apples:** Arrange the apple slices in a single layer on a baking sheet lined with parchment paper. Sprinkle evenly with cinnamon and nutmeg.
   - **British Touch:** Dust the apple slices with sugar-free custard powder before baking. This will give them a creamy, vanilla-like flavor as they bake.
3. **Bake:** Place the baking sheet in the preheated oven and bake for 15-20 minutes, or until the apples are tender and lightly golden.
4. **Serve:** Remove the apple slices from the oven.
   - **American Twist:** Serve the warm apple slices with a dollop of sugar-free whipped cream on top for a luxurious finish.
5. **Enjoy:** Dive into this warm, spiced, and comforting treat, perfect for a dessert or a sweet snack.

Tips and Variations
- **Different Spices:** Experiment with other spices like clove or allspice for different flavor profiles.
- **Additional Toppings:** For extra crunch, add a sprinkle of chopped nuts such as almonds or pecans before baking.

Storage and Serving Suggestions
- **Best Served Fresh:** These baked apple slices are best enjoyed fresh out of the oven while they're still warm and aromatic.
- **Reheating:** If you have leftovers, reheat them in the oven or microwave to restore their warmth before serving.

Nutritional Information per Serving
- **Calories:** 150 kcal - **Protein:** 0.5 g (1% of RDV)
- **Carbohydrates:** 34 g (11%) - **Sugars:** 25 g
- **Fat:** 0 g (0%) - **Saturated Fat:** 0 g (0%)
- **Fiber:** 5 g (20%) - **Sodium:** 10 mg (0.4%)

75. GREEK YOGURT AND STRAWBERRY PARFAIT

 Prep time: 10 minutes   **Cooking time:** No Expected   **Total time:** 10 minutes **Servings:** 1

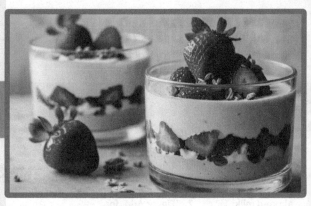

Ingredients

- **Non-fat Greek yogurt:** 1 cup (245 g)
- **Fresh strawberries, hulled and sliced:** 1/2 cup (80 g)
- **Sugar-free granola:** 1/4 cup (30 g)

American Twist:
- **Sugar-free chocolate syrup:** 1 tbsp (15 ml)

British Touch:
- **Sugar-free strawberry jam:** 1 tbsp (15 ml)

Step-by-Step Instructions

1. **Prepare Ingredients:** If not already prepared, hull and slice the strawberries. Set aside a few slices for garnish if desired.
2. **Layer the Parfait:** Begin by spooning a layer of non-fat Greek yogurt into a tall glass or parfait dish.
   - Mix in the sugar-free strawberry jam into half of the Greek yogurt before layering for a **British touch**. This gives a fruity, sweet layer throughout.
3. **Add Strawberries:** Add a layer of sliced strawberries over the yogurt.
4. **Add Granola:** Sprinkle a layer of sugar-free granola over the strawberries. This adds a nice crunch and contrasts beautifully with the creamy texture of the yogurt.
5. **Repeat Layers:** Repeat the layering process, finishing with a top layer of yogurt.
   - **American Twist:** Drizzle sugar-free chocolate syrup over the top layer for a rich, decadent flavor.
6. **Garnish:** Top with the reserved strawberry slices and perhaps a sprinkle of granola or a little more chocolate syrup or strawberry jam, depending on your preference.
7. **Serve:** Enjoy this delicious and nutritious parfait as a healthy breakfast, snack, or dessert.

Tips and Variations
- **Seasonal Berries:** Feel free to add or substitute other berries such as blueberries or raspberries for additional colors and flavors.
- **Protein Boost:** Mix a scoop of protein powder into the yogurt to increase the protein content, perfect for a post-workout snack.

Storage and Serving Suggestions
- **Best Served Fresh:** This parfait is best enjoyed immediately after assembly to maintain the crispness of the granola.
- **Prep Ahead:** If you need to prepare in advance, layer the yogurt and fruit and store in the refrigerator, then add the granola just before serving to keep it crunchy.

Nutritional Information per Serving
- **Calories:** 280 kcal - **Protein:** 20 g (40% of RDV)
- **Carbohydrates:** 35 g (12%) - **Sugars:** 18 g
- **Fat:** 3 g (4.5%) - **Saturated Fat:** 0 g (0%)
- **Fiber:** 4 g (16%) - **Sodium:** 85 mg (3.5%)

76. COCOA AND AVOCADO MOUSSE

 Prep time: 10 minutes   **Cooking time:** No Expected   **Total time:** 10 minutes   **Servings:** 1

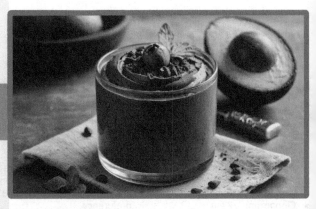

Ingredients

- **Avocado, ripe:** 1 medium (about 200 g)
- **Unsweetened cocoa powder:** 2 tbsps (15 g)
- **Stevia (or another sugar substitute to taste):** 1 tbsp
- **Vanilla extract:** 1 tsp

American Twist:
- **Crushed sugar-free peppermint candies:** 1 tbsp (for topping)

British Touch:
- **Peppermint extract:** 1/4 tsp (mixed in)

Step-by-Step Instructions

1. **Prepare Ingredients:** Halve the avocado, remove the pit, and scoop the flesh into a blender or food processor.
2. **Add Flavorings:** To the avocado, add the unsweetened cocoa powder, stevia, vanilla extract, and **British touch** of peppermint extract. The peppermint extract will infuse the mousse with a refreshing, minty flavor that complements the rich cocoa.
3. **Blend:** Blend the mixture until smooth and creamy. Scrape down the sides as needed to ensure all ingredients are well incorporated.
4. **Serve:** Spoon the mousse into a serving dish or glass.
   - **American Twist:** Top the mousse with crushed sugar-free peppermint candies, adding a crunchy texture and extra minty flavor.
5. **Chill (Optional):** For a firmer texture, chill the mousse in the refrigerator for about 30 minutes before serving.
6. **Enjoy:** Serve this rich and creamy mousse as a delightful and healthy dessert.

Tips and Variations
- **Enhance Creaminess:** For a smoother texture, add a splash of unsweetened almond milk while blending.
- **Extra Toppings:** Garnish with fresh berries or a sprinkle of cocoa powder for an elegant touch.

Storage and Serving Suggestions
- **Best Served Fresh:** This mousse is best enjoyed soon after preparation to preserve the freshness and creamy texture of the avocado.
- **Storage:** If needed, cover and refrigerate for up to one day. Note that the surface may darken slightly due to the avocado's exposure to air.

Nutritional Information per Serving
- **Calories:** 345 kcal - **Protein:** 4 g (8% of RDV)
- **Carbohydrates:** 24 g (8%) - **Sugars:** 1 g
- **Fat:** 27 g (42%) - **Saturated Fat:** 4.5 g (22.5%)
- **Fiber:** 10 g (40%) - **Sodium:** 20 mg (0.8%)

77. ALMOND FLOUR PANCAKES

 Prep time: 10 minutes 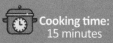 **Cooking time:** 15 minutes   **Total time:** 25 minutes 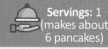 **Servings:** 1 (makes about 6 pancakes)

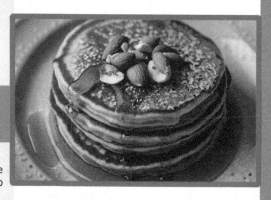

Ingredients

- **Almond flour:** 1 cup (100 g)
- **Eggs:** 2 large
- **Unsweetened almond milk:** 1/2 cup (120 ml)
- **Baking powder:** 1 tsp
- **Salt:** 1/4 tsp
- **Optional:** Sweetener to taste (e.g., stevia or erythritol)

American Twist:

- **Sugar-free maple syrup:** for serving

British Touch:

- **Stewed sugar-free rhubarb:** for serving (prepare by simmering chopped rhubarb with a little water and a sugar substitute until soft and compote-like)

Step-by-Step Instructions

1. **Mix Dry Ingredients:** In a large mixing bowl, combine the almond flour, baking powder, and salt. Mix well to distribute the baking powder evenly.
2. **Add Wet Ingredients:** In another bowl, whisk together the eggs and unsweetened almond milk. If you like your pancakes a bit sweeter, add your chosen sweetener to the wet ingredients.
3. **Combine Mixtures:** Pour the wet ingredients into the dry ingredients and stir until just combined. Be careful not to overmix; a few lumps are okay.
4. **Preheat a Pan:** Heat a non-stick skillet or griddle over medium heat. Lightly grease it with a small amount of butter or oil.
5. **Cook Pancakes:** Pour 1/4 cup of batter for each pancake onto the hot skillet. Cook until bubbles form on the surface and the edges start to look set, about 2-3 minutes. Flip and cook for another 2 minutes or until golden brown and cooked through.
6. **Serve:**
   - **American Twist:** Serve the pancakes with a generous drizzle of sugar-free maple syrup.
   - **British Touch:** Top the pancakes with a spoonful of stewed sugar-free rhubarb for a tangy contrast.

Tips and Variations

- **Flavor Add-ins:** Mix in vanilla extract, cinnamon, or nutmeg into the batter for added flavor.
- **Protein Boost:** Add a scoop of your favorite protein powder to the batter to increase the protein content.

Storage and Serving Suggestions

- **Storage:** Leftover pancakes can be stored in the refrigerator for up to 3 days or frozen for up to a month. Reheat in a toaster or microwave before serving.
- **Make Ahead:** You can mix the dry ingredients in advance and store them in an airtight container. Just add the wet ingredients when you're ready to cook.

Nutritional Information

- **Calories:** 295 kcal - **Protein:** 12 g (24% of RDV)
- **Carbohydrates:** 12 g (4%) - **Sugars:** 2 g
- **Fat:** 23 g (35%) - **Saturated Fat:** 2 g (10%)
- **Fiber:** 6 g (24%) - **Sodium:** 200 mg (8.3%)

78. MATCHA TEA WITH ALMOND MILK

 Prep time: 5 minutes   **Cooking time:** Not Expected   **Total time:** 5 minutes   **Servings:** 1

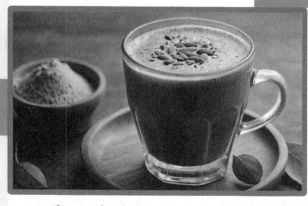

Ingredients

- **Matcha powder:** 1 tsp
- **Almond milk:** 1 cup (240 ml)
- **Natural sweetener (like stevia or honey):** to taste (optional)

American Twist:

- **Vanilla ice cream:** 1 scoop (for blending into a matcha latte)

British Touch:

- **Vanilla extract:** 1/4 tsp (for enhanced flavor)

Step-by-Step Instructions

1. **Prepare Matcha:** Sift the matcha powder into a bowl or cup to remove any clumps. This ensures a smooth tea.
2. **Heat Almond Milk:** Heat the almond milk in a small saucepan over medium heat until hot but not boiling. Alternatively, you can warm it in a microwave.
3. **Whisk:** Add a small amount of the hot almond milk to the matcha powder. Using a matcha whisk or a small regular whisk, vigorously whisk in a "W" motion until the mixture becomes frothy. Add the rest of the almond milk and continue to whisk until the matcha is well dissolved and the beverage is frothy.
   - **Add British Touch:** Stir in a dash of vanilla extract to the matcha tea for a subtly sweet and aromatic flavor, enhancing the natural nuttiness of the almond milk.
4. **Sweeten (Optional):** Sweeten with your choice of natural sweetener to taste, if desired.
   - **American Twist (Matcha Latte):** To make a matcha latte, blend the prepared matcha tea with a scoop of vanilla ice cream in a blender until smooth and creamy. This creates a rich and indulgent version of the traditional matcha latte.
5. **Serve:** If making the traditional matcha with almond milk, serve the beverage hot and frothy.
   - If opting for the American twist, pour the blended matcha latte into a glass and enjoy immediately.

Tips and Variations

- **Cold Version:** For a refreshing summer drink, pour the matcha almond milk over ice and enjoy cold.
- **Enhance Flavor:** Add a sprinkle of cinnamon or nutmeg on top for a spicy finish.

Storage and Serving Suggestions

- **Immediate Consumption:** Best enjoyed immediately after preparation to maintain the flavor and texture, especially when ice cream is involved.

Nutritional Information per Serving

- **Calories:** Approximately 70 kcal (without sweetener and ice cream) - **Protein:** 2 g - **Carbohydrates:** 6 g
- **Sugars:** 0 g (additional sugars depend on the sweetener and ice cream used)
- **Fat:** 4 g - **Fiber:** 1 g - **Sodium:** 100 mg

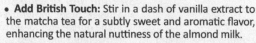

79. PROTEIN GELATIN CUPS

 Prep time: 5 minutes   **Setting time:** 3 hours 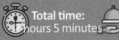 **Total time:** 3 hours 5 minutes **Servings:** 1

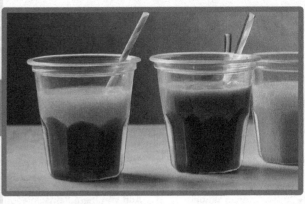

Ingredients

- **Sugar-free gelatin:** 1 packet (about 7 g)
- **Protein powder:** 2 scoops (approximately 60 g)
- **Water:** 2 cups (480 ml)

American Twist:
- Berry-flavored protein powder

British Touch:
- Lemon-flavored protein powder
- Lime zest: 1 tsp

Step-by-Step Instructions

1. **Prepare Gelatin:** In a small saucepan, bring 1 cup (240 ml) of water to a boil. Remove from heat and stir in the sugar-free gelatin until completely dissolved.
2. **Mix Protein Powder:** In a separate bowl, mix the remaining 1 cup (240 ml) of cold water with the protein powder until smooth. Choose berry-flavored protein powder for the **American twist**, or lemon-flavored protein powder for the British touch.
3. **Combine:** Gradually add the gelatin mixture to the protein mixture, stirring constantly to ensure a smooth consistency.

   - **Add British Twist:** If using the British twist, stir in the lime zest to the mixture for a refreshing citrus note.

4. **Pour into Molds:** Pour the mixture into individual gelatin molds or a large dish that can later be cut into cubes.
5. **Refrigerate:** Chill the mixture in the refrigerator for at least 3 hours, or until firm.
6. **Serve:** Once set, unmold the gelatin cups or cut into portions if set in a large dish.
7. **Enjoy:** Serve as a refreshing, protein-packed dessert or snack.

Tips and Variations
- **Enhance Flavor:** Add fresh or frozen berries to the cups before chilling for additional flavor and texture.
- **Sweetener Option:** If desired, sweeten the mixture with a sugar substitute such as stevia or erythritol to enhance the flavor without adding sugar.

Storage and Serving Suggestions
- **Storage:** Protein Gelatin Cups can be stored in the refrigerator for up to 5 days. Keep them covered to prevent them from absorbing odors from other foods.
- **Portable Snack:** These gelatin cups are great for on-the-go snacking or as a post-workout protein boost.

Nutritional Information per Serving
- **Calories:** 120 kcal - **Protein:** 15 g (30% of RDV)
- **Carbohydrates:** 1 g (<1%) - **Sugars:** 0 g
- **Fat:** 1 g (1.5%) - **Saturated Fat:** 0 g (0%)
- **Fiber:** 0 g (0%) - **Sodium:** 100 mg (4.2%)

80. RICOTTA AND BERRY COMPOTE

 Prep time: 10 minutes   **Cook time:** 10 minutes   **Total time:** 20 minutes   **Servings:** 1

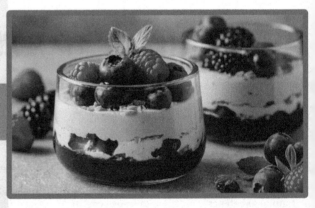

Ingredients

- **Low-fat ricotta cheese:** 1 cup (250 g)
- **Mixed berries (such as strawberries, blueberries, raspberries):** 1 cup (150 g)
- **Sugar substitute (such as stevia or erythritol):** to taste

American Twist:
- Sugar-free cinnamon: 1/4 tsp (for sprinkling)

British Touch:
- Sugar-free clotted cream: 1 tbsp (for topping)

Step-by-Step Instructions

1. **Prepare Berry Compote:** In a small saucepan, combine the mixed berries and sugar substitute. Cook over medium heat, stirring occasionally, until the berries break down and form a compote, about 8-10 minutes. Adjust the sweetness according to taste.

2. **Chill Compote:** Remove the compote from heat and let it cool slightly. For a quicker cool down, place it in the refrigerator for a few minutes.

3. **Assemble Dessert:**

   - **Layer Ricotta:** Spoon the ricotta cheese into two serving bowls or glasses.

4. **Add Compote:** Divide the berry compote evenly and spoon it over the ricotta cheese.

   - **American Twist:** Sprinkle sugar-free cinnamon over the compote for a warm, spiced flavor.
   - **British Touch:** Top each serving with a spoonful of sugar-free clotted cream for a rich, creamy texture.

5. **Serve:** Enjoy this dessert chilled or at room temperature as a delightful end to a meal or as a nutritious snack.

Tips and Variations
- **Enhance Flavor:** Enhance the berry compote with a splash of vanilla extract or a squeeze of fresh lemon juice for added depth.
- **Seasonal Berries:** Use fresh seasonal berries when available for the best flavor and texture.

Storage and Serving Suggestions
- **Storage:** Store any leftover compote in an airtight container in the refrigerator for up to 3 days. The ricotta should also be refrigerated and is best used within 3 days.
- **Make Ahead:** Prepare the berry compote ahead of time and store it in the refrigerator to save on preparation time when serving.

Nutritional Information per Serving
- **Calories:** 180 kcal - **Protein:** 14 g (28% of RDV)
- **Carbohydrates:** 18 g (6%) - **Sugars:** 8 g (natural sugars from berries) - **Fat:** 8 g (12%)
- **Saturated Fat:** 5 g (25%) - **Fiber:** 3 g (12%)
- **Sodium:** 125 mg (5.2%)

DESSERTS

81. PUMPKIN SPICE CUSTARD

 Prep time: 10 minutes   **Cook time:** 30 minutes   **Total time:** 40 minutes   **Servings:** 1

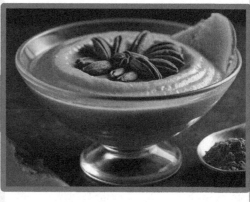

Ingredients
- **Pumpkin puree:** 1 cup (240 g)
- **Eggs:** 2 large
- **Nutmeg:** 1/2 tsp
- **Cinnamon:** 1 tsp
- **Sugar substitute (such as stevia or erythritol):** to taste

American Twist:
- **Sugar-free caramel topping:** for sprinkling

British Touch:
- **Ground cloves:** 1/4 tsp (mixed in)
- **Sugar-free ginger snaps:** for serving

Step-by-Step Instructions
1. **Preheat Oven:** Preheat your oven to 350°F (175°C). Place four ramekins or small baking dishes in a baking pan and set aside.
2. **Prepare Custard Mixture:** In a mixing bowl, whisk together the pumpkin puree, eggs, nutmeg, cinnamon, and sugar substitute until smooth and well combined.

   • **Add British Touch:** Mix in the ground cloves for the British touch, providing a warm and aromatic flavor to the custard.
3. **Divide Mixture:** Pour the custard mixture evenly into the prepared ramekins or baking dishes.
4. **Bake:** Carefully pour hot water into the baking pan to reach halfway up the sides of the ramekins. This creates a water bath, ensuring gentle and even cooking of the custard.
5. **Bake:** Place the baking pan in the preheated oven and bake for 25-30 minutes, or until the custard is set around the edges but slightly wobbly in the center.
6. **Cool:** Remove the custards from the oven and allow them to cool in the water bath for a few minutes before transferring to a wire rack to cool completely.
7. **Chill (Optional):** For a firmer texture, refrigerate the custards for at least 1 hour before serving.
8. **Serve:** Sprinkle each custard with a touch of sugar-free caramel topping for the American twist.
9. **Enjoy:** Serve the pumpkin spice custards with sugar-free ginger snaps on the side for a delightful and satisfying dessert.

Tips and Variations
- **Texture Variation:** For a smoother texture, strain the custard mixture through a fine-mesh sieve before pouring it into the ramekins.
- **Make Ahead:** These custards can be made ahead of time and stored in the refrigerator for up to two days before serving.

Storage and Serving Suggestions
- **Storage:** Store any leftover custards in the refrigerator, tightly covered, for up to three days.
- **Reheating:** To reheat, place the custards in a preheated oven at 325°F (160°C) for about 10 minutes, or until warmed through.

Nutritional Information per Serving
- **Calories:** 90 kcal - **Protein:** 5 g (10% of RDV)
- **Carbohydrates:** 8 g (3%) - **Sugars:** 2 g
- **Fat:** 4 g (6%) - **Saturated Fat:** 1.5 g (7.5%)
- **Fiber:** 2 g (8%) - **Sodium:** 50 mg (2.1%)

82. CHOCOLATE ZUCCHINI BROWNIES

 Prep time: 10 minutes   **Cook time:** 15-20 minutes   **Total time:** 25-30 minutes   **Servings:** 1

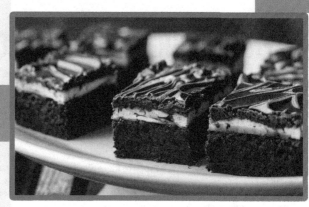

Ingredients
- **Grated zucchini:** 1/4 cup
- **Almond flour:** 1/4 cup
- **Unsweetened cocoa powder:** 2 tbsps
- **Stevia (or another suitable sugar substitute):** to taste (equivalent to 1 tbsp sugar)
- **Egg:** 1 small or 1/2 a large beaten
- **Vanilla extract:** 1/4 tsp
- **Baking powder:** 1/8 tsp
- **Salt:** a pinch

American Twist:
- **Sugar-free peanut butter chips:** 1 tbsp

British Touch:
- **Splash of sugar-free orange essence:** 1/4 tsp

Step-by-Step Instructions
1. **Preheat Oven and Prepare Pan:**

   • Preheat your oven to 350°F (175°C).
   • Grease a small oven-safe dish or a mini baking pan.
2. **Mix Dry Ingredients:** In a mixing bowl, combine the almond flour, unsweetened cocoa powder, stevia, baking powder, and salt.
3. **Add Wet Ingredients:** Stir in the grated zucchini, beaten egg, and vanilla extract.

   • **British Touch:** Add a splash of sugar-free orange essence to the mixture.
4. **Combine Mixtures:** Add the dry ingredients to the wet ingredients and stir until just combined.

   • **American Twist:** Fold in sugar-free peanut butter chips.
5. **Bake:**

   • Pour the batter into the prepared baking dish, smoothing the top with a spatula.
   • Bake in the preheated oven for 15-20 minutes or until a toothpick inserted into the center comes out mostly clean.
6. **Cool and Serve:**

   • Let the brownie cool in the pan for at least 10 minutes before slicing.
   • Serve warm or at room temperature.

Tips and Variations
- **Additional Flavor:** Add a pinch of cinnamon or nutmeg to the batter for extra warmth.
- **Texture Variants:** For nuttier texture and extra protein, add chopped walnuts or pecans.

Nutritional Information
- **Calories:** Approximately 180 kcal - **Protein:** 5 g
- **Carbohydrates:** 15 g - **Sugars:** 1 g
- **Fat:** 12 g - **Fiber:** 3 g
- **Sodium:** 75 mg

83. SUGAR-FREE LEMON BARS

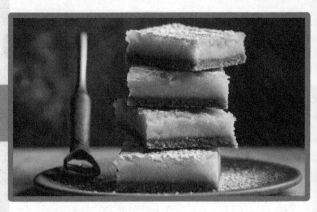

 Prep time: 10 minutes 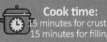 **Cook time:** 15 minutes for crust + 15 minutes for filling   **Total time:** 40 minutes **Servings:** 1

Ingredients

For the Crust:
- **Almond flour:** 3 tbsps
- **Butter, melted:** 1 tbsp
- **Sugar substitute (such as erythritol):** 1 tsp
- **Salt:** a pinch

For the Lemon Filling:
- **Egg:** 1 large
- **Sugar substitute (equivalent to 2 tbsps sugar)**
- **Lemon zest:** From 1/2 lemon
- **Fresh lemon juice:** 1 tbsp

American Twist:
- **Sugar-free powdered sugar:** For dusting

British Touch:
- **Sugar-free blackberry jam:** 1 tsp

Step-by-Step Instructions

1. **Preheat Oven and Prepare Pan:** Preheat your oven to 350°F (175°C). Line a small oven-safe dish or ramekin with parchment paper.
2. **Make the Crust:** In a small bowl, mix the almond flour, melted butter, sugar substitute, and a pinch of salt until well combined. Press the mixture firmly into the bottom of the prepared dish.
3. Bake in the preheated oven for about 15 minutes or until slightly golden. Remove from the oven and let cool slightly.
   - **Add British Touch:** Spread a layer of sugar-free blackberry jam over the cooled crust.
4. **Prepare Lemon Filling:** In a separate bowl, whisk together the egg, sugar substitute, lemon zest, and lemon juice until well blended. Pour this mixture over the blackberry jam layer.
5. **Bake Again:** Return the dish to the oven and bake for an additional 15 minutes, or until the filling is set. Remove from the oven and let cool completely in the pan.
   - **Add American Twist:** Once cooled, sift sugar-free powdered sugar over the top of the lemon bars for a traditional American finish.
6. **Chill and Serve:** Chill the bars in the refrigerator for at least 1 hour to firm up before serving. Cut into the desired shape and serve.

Tips and Variations
- **Citrus Variations:** Consider using lime juice and zest for a twist on the traditional lemon flavor.
- **Texture Additions:** Sprinkle toasted almond slices on top for added crunch and flavor.

Storage and Serving Suggestions
- **Storage:** Store the lemon bar in the refrigerator and consume within 2-3 days for optimal freshness.
- **Serving:** This lemon bar is perfect as a light dessert or an afternoon treat with tea or coffee.

Nutritional Information
- **Calories:** Approximately 250 kcal - **Protein:** 6 g
- **Carbohydrates:** 10 g - **Sugars:** 1 g
- **Fat:** 20 g - **Fiber:** 2 g
- **Sodium:** 200 mg

84. FROZEN GREEK YOGURT POPS

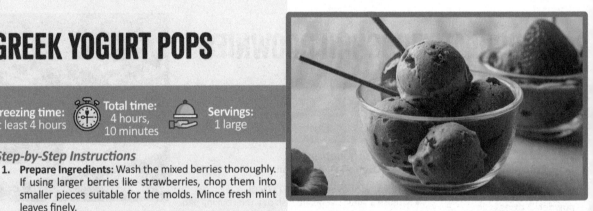

 Prep time: 10 minutes   **Freezing time:** at least 4 hours   **Total time:** 4 hours, 10 minutes   **Servings:** 1 large

Ingredients
- **Non-fat Greek yogurt:** 1/2 cup (120 g)
- **Mixed berries (such as strawberries, blueberries, raspberries):** 1/4 cup (37.5 g)
- **Stevia (or another suitable sugar substitute):** to taste

American Twist:
- **Chopped sugar-free dark chocolate:** 1 tbsp

British Touch:
- **Minced mint:** 1 tbsp

Step-by-Step Instructions

1. **Prepare Ingredients:** Wash the mixed berries thoroughly. If using larger berries like strawberries, chop them into smaller pieces suitable for the molds. Mince fresh mint leaves finely.
2. **Mix the Ingredients:** In a mixing bowl, combine the Greek yogurt, mixed berries, and stevia. Adjust the sweetness according to your preference.
   - **British Touch:** Add the minced mint to the yogurt mixture, mixing well to distribute evenly.
   - **Add American Twist:** Fold in chopped sugar-free dark chocolate into the mixture, ensuring it's evenly distributed throughout the yogurt.
3. **Fill the Molds:** Spoon the yogurt mixture into ice pop molds. Tap the molds gently on the counter to remove any air pockets and ensure the mixture settles properly. Insert sticks into each mold.
4. **Freeze:** Place the molds in the freezer and freeze for at least 4 hours, or until the yogurt pops are completely solid.
5. **Serve:** When ready to serve, run warm water over the outside of the molds for a few seconds to loosen the pops. Gently pull the sticks to release the yogurt pops. Enjoy immediately as a refreshing and healthy treat.

Tips and Variations
- **Flavor Options:** Experiment with other fruit combinations or add pureed fruit for a smoother texture.
- **Protein Boost:** Add a scoop of your favorite protein powder to the yogurt before mixing with other ingredients for an extra protein kick.

Storage and Serving Suggestions
- **Storage:** Keep the frozen yogurt pops in the freezer and consume within 2 weeks for the best quality.
- **Prep Ahead:** These are perfect for making ahead of time for parties or as a go-to cool snack during hot weather.

Nutritional Information per Serving
- **Calories:** Approximately 150 kcal - **Protein:** 10 g
- **Carbohydrates:** 15 g - **Sugars:** 8 g (varies based on the amount of stevia used and the natural sugars in the berries)
- **Fat:** 3 g - **Fiber:** 2 g - **Sodium:** 45 mg

85. ENERGIZING GREEN SMOOTHIE

 Prep time: 5 minutes   **Cooking time:** No Expected   **Total time:** 5 minutes   **Servings:** 1 large

Ingredients

- **Spinach:** 1 cup (30 g)
- **Apple, cored and chopped:** 1 medium
- **Banana, sliced:** 1 medium
- **Celery, chopped:** 1 stalk
- **Coconut water:** 1 cup (240 ml)

American Twist:

- **Protein powder:** 1 scoop (approx. 30 g)

British Touch:

- Additional handful of spinach leaves)

Step-by-Step Instructions

1. **Prepare Ingredients:** Rinse the spinach thoroughly to remove any grit. Core and chop the apple. There is no need to peel it unless you prefer a smoother texture. Peel and slice the banana for easier blending. Chop the celery into small pieces.

2. **Blend the Smoothie:** In a blender, combine the spinach, apple, banana, celery, and coconut water.

   - **Add British Touch:** Add an extra handful of spinach leaves for a deeper green color and enhanced nutritional value.

3. Blend on high until all the ingredients are completely smooth.

   - **Add American Twist:** Add a scoop of your favorite protein powder to the blender. This will help make the smoothie more filling and increase its protein content, which is great for post-workout recovery or a more satisfying meal replacement.

4. Blend again until the protein powder is fully incorporated and the smoothie is smooth.

5. **Serve:** Pour the smoothie into one large glass for a filling meal, or divide it into two smaller glasses if sharing. Enjoy immediately to benefit from the maximum amount of nutrients.

Tips and Variations

- **Ice Cubes:** Add a few ice cubes to the blender if you prefer a colder smoothie or if your ingredients are not chilled.
- **Sweetness Adjustment:** If you find the smoothie needs a bit more sweetness, you can add a little honey or another preferred sweetener to taste.
- **Nutrient Boost:** For an additional nutrient boost, consider adding chia seeds or flaxseeds to the smoothie before blending.

Storage and Serving Suggestions

- **Immediate Consumption:** This smoothie is best enjoyed immediately after blending to take advantage of its freshness and full nutritional benefits.
- **Prep Ahead:** You can prepare the chopped fruits and vegetables ahead of time and keep them in the fridge for quick assembly and blending in the morning.

Nutritional Information per Serving

- **Calories:** Approximately 250 kcal
- **Protein:** 8 g (if using protein powder)
- **Carbohydrates:** 50 g - **Sugars:** 30 g (natural sugars from fruits) - **Fat:** 1 g
- **Saturated Fat:** 0 g - **Fiber:** 8 g - **Sodium:** 150 mg

---

86. CUCUMBER LEMON DETOX WATER

 Prep time: 5 minutes   **Infusion time:** 1-2 hours for flavor integration   **Total time:** 1 hour 5 minutes   **Servings:** 1 large

Ingredients

- **Cucumber:** 1/4 medium cucumber, thinly sliced
- **Lemon:** 1/4 lemon, thinly sliced
- **Fresh mint leaves:** 3-4 leaves
- **Water:** 1 cup (240 ml)

American Twist:

- Freeze some cucumber slices to use as ice cubes

British Touch:

- Substitute lemon juice with elderflower cordial: 1 tbsp

Step-by-Step Instructions

1. **Prepare Ingredients:** Thinly slice the cucumber and lemon. If applying the American twist, place a few cucumber slices in the freezer until they are frozen.

2. **Assemble Ingredients:** In a large glass, combine the fresh cucumber slices (including any frozen ones, if using), lemon slices, and fresh mint leaves.

   - **Add British Touch:** Instead of squeezing the lemon, add elderflower cordial to the glass for a subtle floral sweetness that complements the cucumber.

3. **Add Water:** Fill the glass with water (preferably filtered or sparkling for an extra refreshing touch).

4. **Infuse:** Allow the ingredients to infuse in the refrigerator for at least 1-2 hours. This helps the flavors meld together more profoundly, enhancing the refreshing taste.

5. **Serve:** Once infused, stir gently and enjoy chilled. You can add more fresh mint or a fresh slice of cucumber or lemon for garnish.

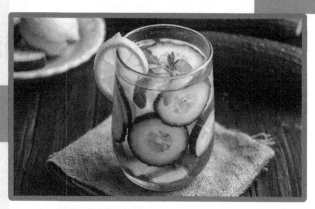

Tips and Variations

- **Enhanced Flavors:** For a stronger infusion, muddle the cucumber and mint slightly before adding the water.
- **Sweetener Option:** If you prefer a slightly sweeter drink, you can add a tsp of honey or another natural sweetener.

Storage and Serving Suggestions

- **Best Served Fresh:** This detox water is best enjoyed within a day of preparation to ensure maximum freshness and flavor.
- **Variety:** Experiment with other hydrating ingredients like watermelon, orange slices, or fresh ginger for different flavor profiles.

Nutritional Information per Serving

- **Calories:** Approx. 15 kcal - **Protein:** 0 g
- **Carbohydrates:** 4 g
- **Sugars:** 2 g (natural sugars from cucumber and elderflower cordial)
- **Fat:** 0 g - **Fiber:** 1 g
- **Sodium:** 2 mg

87. LEMON GINGER GREEN TEA

 Prep time: 5 minutes **Steep time:** 10-15 minutes 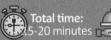 **Total time:** 15-20 minutes **Servings:** 1

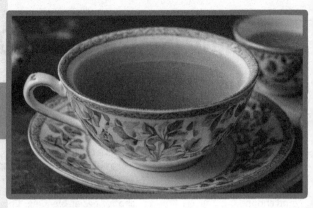

Ingredients
- **Green tea bag:** 1
- **Lemon juice:** From 1/2 a lemon
- **Fresh ginger root:** 1-inch piece, peeled and thinly sliced
- **Water:** 1 cup (240 ml)

American Twist:
- **Honey:** 1 tsp (or to taste)

British Touch:
- Extended steeping time for the ginger root

Step-by-Step Instructions
1. **Prepare Ingredients:**
   - Boil 1 cup of water in a kettle or saucepan.
   - While the water is heating, peel and thinly slice the ginger root.
2. **Steep the Tea:** Place the sliced ginger in the cup first. Pour the hot water directly over the ginger.
   - **British Touch:** Allow the ginger to steep in the hot water for 5-7 minutes before adding the green tea bag. This longer steeping time enhances the ginger's potency and flavor, which is a preferred method in British tea culture.
3. After the ginger has steeped, add the green tea bag and continue to steep the tea for an additional 3-5 minutes, depending on how strong you like your tea.
4. **Add Flavors:** Squeeze the juice from half a lemon into the tea.
   - **American Twist:** Stir in a tsp of honey to sweeten the tea, adding a touch of sweetness that complements the sharpness of the ginger and the tartness of the lemon.
5. **Serve:** Remove the tea bag and ginger slices from the tea, or leave the ginger in for even more flavor as you sip. Serve the tea warm, ensuring it's at a comfortable temperature to drink.

Tips and Variations
- **Cold Version:** This tea can also be enjoyed cold. Simply prepare it in advance, let it cool, and refrigerate. Serve with ice cubes for a refreshing iced tea version.
- **Additional Spices:** For a spicier kick, add a pinch of cayenne pepper or a cinnamon stick during the steeping process.

Storage and Serving Suggestions
- **Immediate Enjoyment:** This tea is best enjoyed immediately after brewing to make the most of the fresh flavors.
- **Storage for Later:** If you have leftovers, store in the refrigerator and consume within 24 hours for the best taste. Reheat gently or enjoy cold.

Nutritional Information per Serving
- **Calories:** Approximately 25 kcal - **Protein:** 0 g
- **Carbohydrates:** 7 g (including honey)
- **Sugars:** 6 g (natural sugars from honey and lemon)
- **Fat:** 0 g - **Fiber:** 0 g
- **Sodium:** 5 mg

88. ANTIOXIDANT BERRY SMOOTHIE

 Prep time: 10 minutes **Cooking time:** Not Expected **Total time:** 10 minutes **Servings:** 1 large

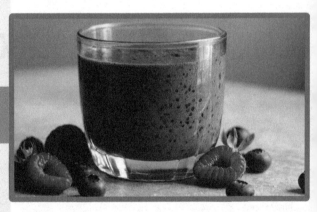

Ingredients
- **Blueberries:** 1/2 cup (70 g)
- **Raspberries:** 1/2 cup (60 g)
- **Strawberries, hulled:** 1/2 cup (75 g)
- **Greek yogurt:** 1/2 cup (120 g)
- **Chia seeds:** 1 tbsp (15 g)

American Twist:
- **Granola:** 2 tbsps (for topping)

British Touch:
- **Low-fat clotted cream:** 1 tbsp (for blending)

Step-by-Step Instructions
1. **Prepare Ingredients:** Wash the blueberries, raspberries, and strawberries thoroughly. Hull the strawberries and cut into halves if they are large. Measure out the Greek yogurt and chia seeds.
2. **Blend the Smoothie:** In a blender, combine the blueberries, raspberries, strawberries, Greek yogurt, and chia seeds.
   - **British Touch:** Add a dollop of low-fat clotted cream to the blender. This will give the smoothie a richer, creamier texture, enhancing its luxurious feel.
   - Blend on high until the mixture is smooth and creamy. If the smoothie is too thick, you can add a little water or more Greek yogurt to reach your desired consistency.
   - **Add American Twist:** Once blended, pour the smoothie into a serving glass or divide it between two glasses.
3. **Serve:** Top each serving with a sprinkle of granola for a delightful crunch and added fiber. Enjoy this antioxidant-packed smoothie immediately to take advantage of its fresh flavors and nutritional benefits.

Tips and Variations
- **Extra Nutrition:** For additional antioxidants and a nutritional boost, consider adding a handful of spinach or kale to the smoothie before blending. These greens won't significantly alter the taste but will enhance the health benefits.
- **Vegan Option:** For a vegan version, substitute the Greek yogurt with a plant-based yogurt such as almond or coconut yogurt, and ensure the granola is vegan if using.

Storage and Serving Suggestions
- **Immediate Consumption:** This smoothie is best enjoyed fresh right after blending to ensure maximum flavor and nutrient intake.
- **Prep Ahead:** If you're short on time in the mornings, you can prepare the fruits the night before and store them in the fridge. Just blend with yogurt and chia seeds when ready to serve.

Nutritional Information per Serving
- **Calories:** Approximately 300 kcal - **Protein:** 12 g
- **Carbohydrates:** 45 g - **Sugars:** 25 g (natural sugars from fruits)
- **Fat:** 8 g - **Saturated Fat:** 3 g
- **Fiber:** 8 g - **Sodium:** 50 mg

89. WATERMELON MINT INFUSED WATER

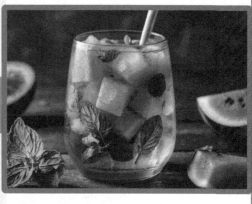

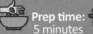 **Prep time:** 5 minutes
 Infusion time: 30 minutes to 1 hour for enhanced flavors
 Total time: 35 minutes to 1 hour, 5 minutes
Servings: 1

Ingredients:
- **Fresh watermelon:** 1/2 cup, cubed
- **Fresh mint leaves:** 3-4 leaves
- **Lime juice:** 1 tbsp (omit for British touch)
- **Water:** 1 cup (240 ml)
- **Ice cubes** (optional)

American Twist:
- Freeze some watermelon chunks to use as ice cubes

British Touch:
- Substitute lime juice with elderflower cordial: 1 tbsp

Step-by-Step Instructions
1. **Prepare Ingredients:** Cube the watermelon into small bite-sized pieces. If applying the American twist, place a portion of the watermelon cubes in the freezer until they are frozen solid. Wash and gently pat dry the mint leaves.
2. **Assemble Ingredients:** In a large glass or mason jar, add the fresh watermelon cubes (including any frozen ones, if using) and fresh mint leaves.
3. **Add Lime Juice or British Touch:** If making the standard version, squeeze in the lime juice over the watermelon and mint.

   • **British Touch:** Instead of lime juice, pour elderflower cordial into the glass for a lovely floral flavor that complements the freshness of watermelon and mint.
4. **Add Water and Ice:** Fill the glass with cold water. Add ice cubes if desired for an extra chill.
5. **Infuse:** Allow the ingredients to infuse by placing the glass in the refrigerator for at least 30 minutes to 1 hour. This helps the flavors to meld together, creating a more refreshing drink.
6. **Serve:** Stir gently before serving. Enjoy this refreshing infused water chilled, straight from the glass.

Tips and Variations
- **Enhanced Flavor:** For a more intense flavor, muddle the mint leaves and watermelon slightly before adding the water.
- **Additional Flavors:** Consider adding other fruits like cucumber slices or berries for additional flavor layers.

Storage and Serving Suggestions
- **Immediate Consumption:** Best enjoyed within a few hours of preparation to enjoy the freshness of the ingredients.
- **Outdoor Events:** Ideal for taking along to picnics or outdoor events in a sealed bottle or jar.

Nutritional Information per Serving
- **Calories:** Approx. 30 kcal - **Protein:** 0 g
- **Carbohydrates:** 7 g - **Sugars:** 6 g (natural sugars from watermelon and elderflower cordial)
- **Fat:** 0 g - **Fiber:** 0.5 g - **Sodium:** 3 mg

---

90. GOLDEN MILK

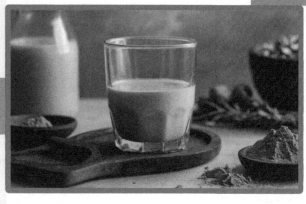

 Prep time: 2 minutes
 Cook time: 5 minutes
 Total time: 7 minutes
 Servings: 1

Ingredients
- **Almond milk:** 1 cup (240 ml)
- **Turmeric powder:** 1/2 tsp
- **Ginger, fresh and grated:** 1/4 tsp
- **Honey:** 1 tsp (adjust based on taste preference)
- **Black pepper:** A pinch (to enhance turmeric absorption)

American Twist:
- **Cayenne pepper:** A pinch (for added heat and metabolism boost)

British Touch:
- **Ground cardamom:** A pinch (for a sweet, aromatic flavor)

Step-by-Step Instructions
1. **Heat Ingredients:** In a small saucepan, combine the almond milk, turmeric powder, grated ginger, and a pinch of black pepper.

   • **British Touch:** Add a pinch of ground cardamom along with the other spices. This will impart a subtle, aromatic sweetness that complements the earthy turmeric and spicy ginger.
2. **Simmer:** Place the saucepan over low to medium heat. Allow the mixture to gently simmer — do not boil — for about 5 minutes. This will help the flavors to meld and ensure the ginger and turmeric are well infused.

   • **Add Sweetener and American Twist:** After simmering, remove from heat. Stir in the honey to sweeten the mixture.
   • **American Twist:** Add a pinch of cayenne pepper here if desired. This will introduce a spicy kick that enhances the warming effect of the drink.
3. **Serve:** Pour the golden milk into a mug through a strainer to remove the pieces of ginger.

4. Serve the golden milk warm, ensuring it's at a comfortable temperature to drink.

Tips and Variations
- **Vegan Option:** Ensure the honey is substituted with agave syrup or another vegan sweetener if serving to those avoiding animal products.
- **Enhanced Flavor:** For a deeper flavor, you can toast the dry spices in the saucepan for a minute before adding the milk.
- **Creamier Texture:** Use full-fat coconut milk in place of almond milk for a richer, creamier texture.

Storage and Serving Suggestions
- **Immediate Consumption:** Golden milk is best enjoyed immediately while warm.
- **Reheating:** If you need to reheat the golden milk, do so gently on the stove to avoid boiling, which can degrade some of the beneficial properties of the ingredients.

Nutritional Information per Serving
- **Calories:** Approximately 60 kcal - **Protein:** 1 g
- **Carbohydrates:** 9 g - **Sugars:** 6 g (from honey)
- **Fat:** 2.5 g - **Saturated Fat:** 0 g
- **Fiber:** 0.5 g - **Sodium:** 50 mg

 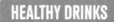

91. HIBISCUS MINT TEA

 Prep time: 5 minutes   **Steep time:** 5-10 minutes 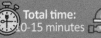 **Total time:** 10-15 minutes **Servings:** 1

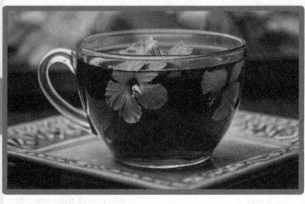

Ingredients:
- **Dried hibiscus flowers:** 1 tbsp
- **Fresh mint leaves:** 4-5 leaves
- **Hot water:** 1 cup (240 ml)

American Twist:

- **Cranberry juice:** 1 tbsp (for adding to the tea)

British Touch:

- **Stevia:** To taste (for sweetening)

Step-by-Step Instructions
1. **Prepare Ingredients:** Boil 1 cup of water in a kettle or pot.

2. **Steep the Tea:** In a large teacup or a heatproof glass, place the dried hibiscus flowers and fresh mint leaves.

3. **Pour the hot water** over the hibiscus and mint. Allow it to steep for 5-10 minutes, depending on how strong you prefer your tea. The longer it steeps, the more intense the flavors and the deeper the color.

   - **Add British Touch:** If you prefer a sweeter tea, sweeten with stevia to taste while the tea is hot. This allows the natural sweetener to dissolve thoroughly.
   - **Add American Twist:** Just before serving, add a splash of cranberry juice to the tea for a tart, fruity flavor that complements the tanginess of the hibiscus.

4. **Serve:** Stir the tea to mix in the sweetener and cranberry juice evenly. Enjoy the tea hot, or let it cool down and serve over ice for a refreshing iced tea option.

Tips and Variations
- **Cold Version:** This tea is also delicious served cold. Refrigerate for a few hours and serve over ice for a refreshing summer beverage.
- **Additional Flavors:** Experiment by adding other herbs such as lemongrass or spices like cinnamon or ginger during the steeping process for added complexity.

Storage and Serving Suggestions
- **Best Served Fresh:** While this tea can be refrigerated and consumed cold, it is best enjoyed fresh for the most vibrant flavors.
- **Make Ahead:** You can steep the tea and store it in the refrigerator overnight, adding cranberry juice and sweetener just before serving.

Nutritional Information per Serving
- **Calories:** Approx. 10 kcal (without stevia) - **Protein:** 0 g
- **Carbohydrates:** 2 g - **Sugars:** 1 g (from cranberry juice)
- **Fat:** 0 g - **Fiber:** 0 g
- **Sodium:** 0 mg

92. TROPICAL SMOOTHIE

 Prep time: 5 minutes   **Cooking time:** Not Expected   **Total time:** 5 minutes   **Servings:** 1

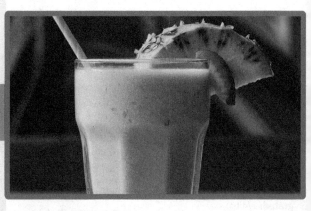

Ingredients
- **Mango:** 1/2 cup, cubed
- **Pineapple:** 1/2 cup, cubed
- **Coconut milk:** 1/2 cup (120 ml)
- **Ice cubes:** 1/2 cup

American Twist:

- **Frozen banana:** 1/2 of a medium banana

British Touch:

- **Pineapple juice:** 1/4 cup (60 ml)

Step-by-Step Instructions
1. **Prepare Ingredients:** Peel and cube the mango and pineapple. If using fresh banana, peel and slice it, then freeze beforehand.

2. **Blend the Smoothie:** In a blender, combine the cubed mango, pineapple, coconut milk, and ice cubes.

   - **American Twist:** Add the frozen banana to the blender. This will give the smoothie a creamy texture and naturally sweet flavor.
   - **British Touch:** Pour in the pineapple juice. This will enhance the tropical flavor and add a little extra sweetness and tartness.

3. **Blend Until Smooth:** Blend on high until all the ingredients are smooth and creamy. If the smoothie is too thick, you can adjust the consistency by adding a little more coconut milk or pineapple juice.

4. **Serve:** Pour the smoothie into a tall glass. Serve immediately for the best taste and texture.

Tips and Variations
- **Enhance the Flavor:** Add a pinch of ground cinnamon or vanilla extract for an extra layer of flavor.
- **Protein Boost:** For a more filling smoothie, add a scoop of your favorite protein powder before blending.

Storage and Serving Suggestions
- **Immediate Consumption:** This smoothie is best enjoyed fresh right after blending to maximize the freshness of the fruits and the creamy texture.

Nutritional Information per Serving
- **Calories:** Approximately 200 kcal
- **Protein:** 2 g
- **Carbohydrates:** 30 g
- **Sugars:** 20 g
- **Fat:** 10 g
- **Fiber:** 3 g
- **Sodium:** 15 mg

HEALTHY DRINKS

93. STRAWBERRY BASIL INFUSED WATER

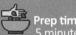 **Prep time:** 5 minutes
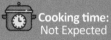 **Cooking time:** Not Expected
 Infusion time: 30 mins to 1 hour
 Total time: 35 minutes to 1 hour 5 minutes

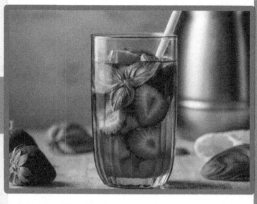

Ingredients

- **Fresh strawberries:** 1/4 cup, sliced
- **Fresh basil leaves:** 3-4 leaves
- **Sparkling water:** 1 cup (240 ml)

American Twist:
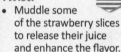
- Muddle some of the strawberry slices to release their juice and enhance the flavor.

British Touch:
- Add a sprig of rosemary to introduce a fragrant, herbal note.

Step-by-Step Instructions

1. **Prepare Ingredients:** Wash the strawberries and basil leaves thoroughly. Slice the strawberries, and gently pat the basil leaves dry.

2. **Assemble Ingredients:** Place the sliced strawberries and basil leaves in a large glass or mason jar.

   - **American Twist:** Muddle some of the strawberry slices in the bottom of the glass before adding the rest. This will release their juices and intensify the flavor of the water.
   - **British Touch:** Add a sprig of rosemary to the glass. This will impart a distinctive, aromatic quality that complements the sweetness of the strawberries.

3. **Add Water:** Pour sparkling water over the strawberries, basil, and rosemary. The carbonation adds a pleasant texture to the infused water.

4. **Infuse:** Allow the mixture to infuse in the refrigerator for at least 30 minutes to 1 hour. The longer it infuses, the more pronounced the flavors.

5. **Serve:** Stir gently before serving to distribute the flavors evenly. Enjoy the infused water chilled, straight from the glass.

Tips and Variations

- **Enhanced Flavor:** For a sweeter drink, you can add a splash of natural sweetener like stevia or honey.
- **Additional Flavors:** Experiment by adding other fruits like lime or cucumber for added complexity.

Storage and Serving Suggestions

- **Best Served Fresh:** This infused water is best enjoyed within a few hours of preparation to enjoy the maximum freshness and effervescence of the sparkling water.
- **Outdoor Refreshment:** Ideal for taking along to picnics or outdoor events in a sealed bottle or jar.

Nutritional Information per Serving

- **Calories:** Approx. 10 kcal - **Protein:** 0 g
- **Carbohydrates:** 2 g
- **Sugars:** 1 g (natural sugars from strawberries)
- **Fat:** 0 g - **Fiber:** 0.5 g - **Sodium:** 10 mg

Dr. Nowzaradan Diet Plan:
30 DAY MEAL PLAN

MEAL PLAN - WEEK 1

DAY	BREAKFAST	SNACK	LUNCH	SNACK	DINNER
MONDAY	Spinach and Blueberry Protein Smoothie	Greek Yogurt with Berries	Chicken Caesar Salad	Apple Slices with Almond Butter	Grilled Chicken with Asparagus
TUESDAY	Oat and Banana Pancakes	Chia Seed Pudding	Beef andw Broccoli Bowl	Baked Kale Chips	Vegetable Lasagna
WEDNESDAY	Avocado and Baked Egg Toast	Cottage Cheese with Pineapple	Tofu Stir-Fry	Edamame Pods	Turkey Shepherd's Pie
THURSDAY	Greek Yogurt with Nuts	Vegetable Sticks with Hummus	Chickpea and Quinoa Salad	Hard-Boiled Eggs	Lentil and Spinach Soup
FRIDAY	Ricotta and Fruit Cream with Nuts	Apple Slices with Almond Butter	Tuna Stuffed Tomato	Roasted Chickpeas	Chicken and Broccoli Bake
SATURDAY	Chia and Berry Smoothie Bowl	Baked Kale Chips	Vegetable Frittata	Greek Yogurt with Berries	Pork and Asparagus Stir-Fry
SUNDAY	Cinnamon Oatmeal Porridge	Chia Seed Pudding	Turkey and Cranberry Wrap	Apple Slices with Almond Butter	Seafood Chowder

MEAL PLAN - WEEK 2

DAY	BREAKFAST	SNACK	LUNCH	SNACK	DINNER
MONDAY	Turkey and Spinach Frittata	Hard-Boiled Eggs	Beef and Vegetable Broth	Baked Kale Chips	Beef Stir-Fry with Snap Peas
TUESDAY	Whole Grain Apple Muffins	Greek Yogurt with Berries	Vegetable Frittata	Edamame Pods	Salmon and Spinach Quiche
WEDNESDAY	Herb Omelette with Bell Peppers	Chia Seed Pudding	Shrimp and Avocado Salad	Vegetable Sticks with Hummus	Lentil and Spinach Soup
THURSDAY	Oat and Banana Bars	Apple Slices with Almond Butter	Turkey and Cranberry Wrap	Roasted Chickpeas	Chicken and Broccoli Bake
FRIDAY	Cinnamon Oatmeal Porridge	Cottage Cheese with Pineapple	Chickpea and Quinoa Salad	Chia Seed Pudding	Pork and Asparagus Stir-Fry
SATURDAY	Chia and Berry Smoothie Bowl	Greek Yogurt with Berries	Chickpea Salad Sandwich	Cucumber and Turkey Roll-ups	Vegetable Lasagna
SUNDAY	Avocado and Baked Egg Toast	Roasted Chickpeas	Turkey and Avocado Salad	Apple Slices with Almond Butter	Turkey Shepherd's Pie

MEAL PLAN - WEEK 3

DAY	BREAKFAST	SNACK	LUNCH	SNACK	DINNER
MONDAY	Whole Grain Apple Muffins	Chia Seed Pudding	Turkey and Avocado Salad	Cottage Cheese with Pineapple	Grilled Tofu Steaks with Zucchini Ribbons
TUESDAY	Oat and Banana Pancakes	Greek Yogurt with Berries	Seafood Chowder	Edamame Pods	Salmon and Spinach Quiche
WEDNESDAY	Ricotta and Fruit Cream with Nuts	Hard-Boiled Eggs	Shrimp and Avocado Salad	Apple Slices with Almond Butter	Turkey Shepherd's Pie
THURSDAY	Cinnamon Oatmeal Porridge	Baked Kale Chips	Beef and Broccoli Bowl	Vegetable Sticks with Hummus	Chicken and Broccoli Bake
FRIDAY	Greek Yogurt with Nuts	Roasted Chickpeas	Vegan Chili	Cucumber and Turkey Roll-ups	Tofu and Vegetable Stir-Fry
SATURDAY	Herb Omelette with Bell Peppers	Chia Seed Pudding	Greek Salad with Chicken	Apple Slices with Almond Butter	Beef Skewers with Bell Peppers
SUNDAY	Egg and Vegetable Casserole	Greek Yogurt with Berries	Seitan and Pepper Skewers	Hard-Boiled Eggs	Hard-Boiled Eggs

MEAL PLAN - WEEK 4

DAY	BREAKFAST	SNACK	LUNCH	SNACK	DINNER
MONDAY	Chia and Berry Smoothie Bowl	Hard-Boiled Eggs	Turkey Casserole	Edamame Pods	Pork and Asparagus Stir-Fry
TUESDAY	Greek Yogurt with Nuts	Baked Kale Chips	Lentil Tomato Soup	Cucumber and Turkey Roll-ups	Beef Skewers with Bell Peppers
WEDNESDAY	Oat and Banana Bars	Apple Slices with Almond Butter	Chickpea Salad Sandwich	Chia Seed Pudding	Vegetable Lasagna
THURSDAY	Avocado and Baked Egg Toast	Cottage Cheese with Pineapple	Grilled Veggie Sandwich	Greek Yogurt with Berries	Salmon and Spinach Quiche
FRIDAY	Egg and Vegetable Casserole	Roasted Chickpeas	Tuna and Bean Salad	Vegetable Sticks with Hummus	Tofu and Vegetable Stir-Fry
SATURDAY	Turkey and Spinach Frittata	Greek Yogurt with Berries	Tuna Stuffed Tomato	Edamame Pods	Turkey Shepherd's Pie
SUNDAY	Cinnamon Oatmeal Porridge	Zucchini Chips	Vegan Chili	Chia Seed Pudding	Lentil and Spinach Soup

This meal plan is structured to provide balanced nutrition with a variety of flavors and ingredients from the "Diet by Dr. Nowzaradan." For those looking to extend this regimen, this plan can be repeated for 90 days, ensuring to adjust meals as necessary to meet personal dietary needs and preferences.

Notes: Portion sizes should be adjusted to meet the 1200 calorie per day target while considering the specific calorie content of each recipe. **Hydration:** It's crucial to drink plenty of water throughout the day to stay hydrated and support metabolic health. **Flexibility:** Feel free to swap similar meals from different days to suit preferences and availability of ingredients while maintaining calorie targets.

GET YOUR FREE BOOK BONUSES NOW!

(DOWNLOAD FOR FREE WITH THE BELOW INSTRUCTION!)

DO YOU WANT EXCLUSIVE BONUSES TO UNLOCK THE FULL KNOWLEDGE ABOUT YOUR DR.NOWZARADAN DIET BOOK?

1) **BONUS 1:** Weight Loss Tracking Journal (Print or Use on your Tablet/Phone)

2) **BONUS 2:** Complete Shopping List

3) **BONUS 3:** Rock-Solid Mindset: No More Discouragement! 10 Phrases to Stay Motivated (READ THEM DAILY!)

SCAN THE QR CODE BELOW AND UNLOCK THE FULL POTENTIAL OF DR. NOWZARADAN DIET BOOK!

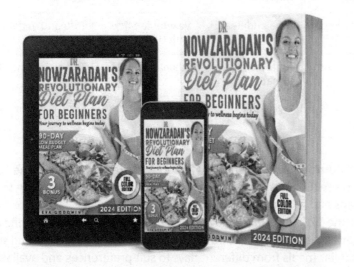

SCAN ME!

INDEX OF INGREDIENTS

INDEX OF INGREDIENTS

Made in the USA
Monee, IL
11 September 2024

65568248R00044